CONFIDENT BREASTFEEDING

ANSHU ARORA

CONFIDENT BREASTFEEDING

Perfect Food For A Perfect Baby

GOOD TIMES BOOKS PVT. LTD.
New Delhi (India)
www.goodtimesbooks.com

Published by

Good Times Books Pvt. Ltd.

H-13, Bali Nagar, New Delhi-110 015 (INDIA)

Phones: +91-11-25913301, 45069086 *Fax:* +91-11-45069086

Email : info@goodtimesbooks.com

Website : www.goodtimesbooks.com

First Published 2011

ISBN-13 : 978-93-806192-2-4

Cataloging in Publication Data--DK

Courtesy: D.K. Agencies (P) Ltd.

<docinfo@dkagencies.com>

Arora, Anshu.

Confident Breastfeeding : perfect food for a perfect baby / Anshu Arora.

p. cm.

ISBN 9789380619224 (pbk.)

1. Breastfeeding. 2. Infants--Nutrition. 3. Mother and child. I. Title.

DDC 649.33 22

Printed in India at

Salasar Imaging Systems

CONTENTS

PREFACE

Over the years there have been several attempts to adopt breastfeeding as the ideal mode of providing nourishment for new born babies in their infancy. At last one can see glimmerings of hope for this very safe and immensely satisfying means of feeding babies and keeping them healthy. Hopefully the idea will catch on at all levels and pave the way for a healthier generation of newborns.

Looking at it anew, breastfeeding seems to be the perfect answer to rich and poor alike who are concerned about the health and wellbeing of their babies. What one marvels at is the manner in which Mother Nature has endowed mothers to be with this priceless gift of breast milk exactly when it is required, in adequate quantities and comprising everything that is necessary for a newborn. What is more, it is available on tap enriched with the right ingredients and at the right temperature. All that the mother has to do is to offer it to her baby as soon as it is born.

In between generations several manufactures of baby food, in particular, of milk powder made it appear that such foods were at an advantage when it came to nourishment for infants. Advertisements made them attractive and their adoption by the upper classes made them even more so.

For today's generation, "going back to Nature" also calls for adopting natural methods to feed one's babies. Breastfeeding is the perfect answer for mother and child. One hopes the message conveyed by this small volume will spread far and wide for the benefit of the coming generation.

...1...

BREASTFEEDING - A MUST FOR BABIES

Breastfeeding is the stage, rather the phenomenon, almost every one of us passes through in the early days of life. It is in fact entry to this world welcomed with the breast milk of mom. There are no set rules about breastfeeding but by watching it frequently, the same can be combined as an art and a science.

Initially you are bound to have problems while you start breastfeeding your newly born baby because none of your friends and relatives have trained you for that. All that you have learnt only by watching a mother breastfeeding her baby during your pregnancy which is the most important and helpful thing you can do to make breastfeeding easier.

It has been seen that the mothers of today do not want to breastfeed because they have to go back to work so soon. It is really shameful on their part for not looking forward to be mothers and for depriving their babies of the best nutritive values that breast milk contains.

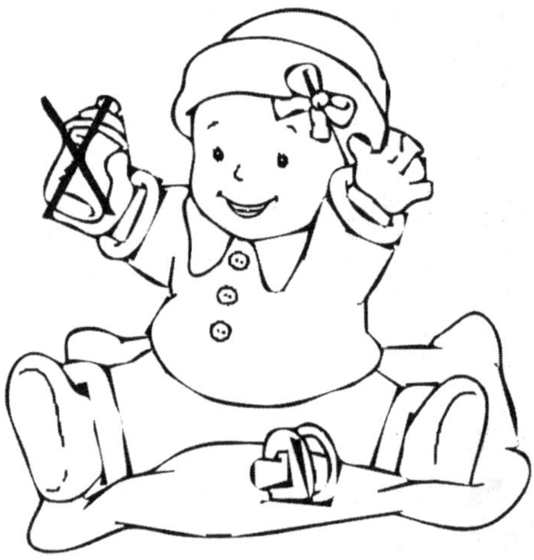

In the olden days of your great grand-mother, women had a good deal of knowledge about breastfeeding and care of babies. Most of the time, there used to be a relative with a new born baby and children moving around to learn how mother helped the baby, changed it, bathed and dressed it, wrapped and fed it. They listened to an experienced relative or any one talking about baby care. All that proved useful for them when they grew up and became mothers. But now things have changed with hospital delivery of babies and rules controlling breastfeeding.

Many successful mothers will tell you that

breastfeeding is not always that easy. It is often a lot harder than most women expect particularly in the early days. You, in fact, get a chance to learn to teach yourself to cope with the problems.

When the baby is born, the midwife and doctor of the hospital along with friends and relatives give their advice about feeding the baby. Though these masses offer their help and support it has been observed that most of them have forgotten the basics of successful breastfeeding. Because of this confusion, some self-help organisations have come into existence providing the necessary guidance to young mothers who breast feed their children These groups have also been trained as breastfeeding counsellors. They render help on the phone and on-line as well.

Essence: Breastfeeding is an art as well as a science.

Dos

1. Learn breastfeeding by watching a mother breastfeeding her baby during your pregnancy.
2. Consult a doctor in case of confusion you have in mind.

Don'ts

1. Deprive your baby of breastfeeding by going back to work very soon.
2. Abide by sayings of the general public.

···2···

BREAST MILK: INGREDIENTS

Breast milk has been considered as the perfect food with numerous advantages such as, it is at the right temperature, bacteria free, containing exactly what your baby needs and even a cat can not reach it. Besides the same comes in attractive containers.

The basic substances of all the kinds of milk are water, proteins, fats, carbohydrates, minerals, vitamins and anti-infective characteristics. The only differences occur as these substances are present in different amounts and varying proportions. Out of these substances each one is different from the next. The proteins of breast milk differ from woman to woman.

The following are the ingredients of breast milk

described briefly. The liquid part of the milk is water with other constituents dissolved in it making its appearance white or creamy depending upon the proportions of various substances present. Water is very important in every part of the body. Lack of it causes dehydration or even death. A dehydrated baby risks getting brain damage.

Breast milk has the right proportions of water and other constituents. It is, therefore, considered as the perfect food for human babies. Many mothers are worried about their milk being dilute. It is very difficult to judge the nutrient value of breast milk by just looking at it. Yellow breast milk is in no way superior to thin bluish white milk.

A thirsty baby when given breast milk gets the right amount of water to satisfy its thirst. If the baby is getting enough breast milk, it need not be given water. In hot weather, the mother has to consume more water and not the baby. Stools of breastfed babies contain more water and hence they never get constipated.

More than one per cent of the breast milk is protein which is made up of curd protein (casein) and whey proteins (lactalbumin and lactoglobulin). Breast milk protein forms finely separated curds in the stomach that pass quickly and easily through the small intestine breaking down without any difficulty. That means the stomach of a breast fed baby empties more quickly.

This is why it gets hungry frequently and needs feeds at short intervals.

Milk contains fat both in saturated and unsaturated forms but breast milk has a higher milk content and contains some lipase of its own that relies solely on lipase in the baby's intestine for its digestion. The fat present in breast milk begins to digest by milk lipase even before it reaches the gut.

Fat is, of course, necessary for the development of the baby particularly for outer coatings of the nerves. The pattern of fatty acids in breast milk has developed in a way to supply the rapidly growing brain and nerves with right building materials at the right time of early infancy. In this time, the tissues grow faster than at any other time.

The bifidus factor is the carbohydrate present in breast milk which acts as very valuable protection against infection in the gut. Purest milk also contains some other sugars which are almost completely absent in cow's milk.

Breast milk comprises some minerals which are important for the health of the baby. Sodium level in breast milk is ideal for human babies. Iron is the mineral present in larger amounts in breast milk.

The latest research shows that iron in breast milk is better absorbed into the blood stream. Vitamins C,

E and copper which are present in higher amounts in breast milk help iron to be absorbed more efficiently.

Breast milk contains vitamins A, C and E. Exclusively breast fed babies do not need any vitamin supplements in the first six months of life. Vitamins in the form of additional foods necessary for the baby should be given to the mother and not the baby. The mother will pass all nutrients through her breast milk in desired proportions to the baby.

There are many substances which also help fight infection in the baby. Many are more plentiful and active in breast milk than in cow's milk.

Essence: Breast milk has unique benefits such as it is always at right temperature, bacteria free, containing what your baby needs, comes in cute containers where even a cat can not reach.

Dos

You have to consume more water in hot weather which will automatically be passed on to the baby via the breast.

Dont's

Give anything other than breast milk for six months initially as it comprises all required nutrients.

…3…

BREAST MILK GOOD FOR MOM AND BABY

While scrutinizing the plus and minus points of breastfeeding we have moved to all aspects and have come to the conclusion that there are no disadvantages of breastfeeding. So to say, the weighing scale falls heavily on the side of 'pros' which means it has the advantages only. If at all breast feeders have any problems, these are easily overcome.

How baby is benefited

Scientifically, breast fed babies have evidence of numerous medical advantages. If the mothers understand the advantages to their babies being breast fed then the pressurefromtheir side will do more than anything to change the poor standard of help as well as advice available to most feeding women in this country.

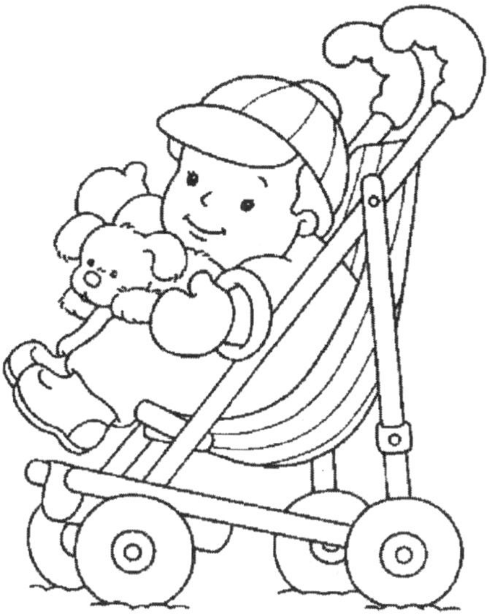

It is perfect food for perfect growth

The unique composition of breast milk doesn't simply provide foodstuff, the amounts of nutrients in breast milk are perfectly geared to the optimum rate of growth of the brain of the baby.

Low infection risk

Breast milk comprising many contents protect a baby from infection caused by bacteria, viruses, yeast and other organisms. In various surveys conducted for babies under six months admitted to hospitals with gastro-enteritis and for respiratory infections, it was observed that only one per cent of the babies were being breast fed. Moreover, it was also seen that bottle fed babies had twice the chances of dying as breast fed babies had.

Fewer allergic diseases

It has been known that eczema, asthma and fever are less common in children who have been breast fed whereas other illnesses are caused by allergy to cow's milk proteins that pass through the gut wall of bottle fed babies

Other plus points for baby

Research has shown that about 80 per cent of fat babies become fat adults but statistically, it has been seen that the breastfed babies rarely face the problem of obesity. Fat people are more prone to heart disease, high blood pressure, diabetes, gallstones and have a reduced life expectancy.

The breast fed baby is less likely to suffer from dental decay as compared to the bottle fed baby. Several specialists report that they see fewer problems of family jaw and mouth development in breast fed babies.

It is interesting to note that studies have shown that breast fed babies walk earlier than bottle fed babies in spite of differences in weight between the two groups and in babies whose mothers went out to work. Moreover, breast fed babies have better IQ than bottle fed ones.

Breast milk contains enough calories providing the right kind of proteins, fats, lactose besides vitamins, iron, minerals, water and enzymes in the amounts necessary for your baby. It also comprises substances preventing harmful bacteria from growing in intestines causing loose motions.

Breast milk is always ready to serve whenever baby wants it needing no preparation. It is at the right temperature, economical, free from contamination and comes in cute containers. Breastfeeding enhances the emotional relationship between child and mother providing warmth, love and affection which is more than food. It also helps in developing brain growth of the baby.

Breast milk is all that baby needs for the first six months. It is easily and quickly digestible also containing immunoglobulins necessary for growth of your baby. Breastfeeding lowers health care costs thereby reducing chances of illness and mortality of children under five years of age. Ultimately it provides budget relief to the family.

How you are benefited

While the mother breast feeds her baby, she feels

that the right thing is done for the baby thereby getting a lot of satisfaction. This act of satisfaction really makes her greatly pleased.

The enjoyment of breastfeeding gives her fulfillment representing the female part of her character. Breast fed babies have more attachment with the mother and she is three times as likely to sleep with them as against bottle feeders.

Three months after delivery, she is more likely to lose weight without dieting than the mother who is bottle feeding. Breastfeeding helps the mother to get back to pre-pregnancy shape and weight. If the shape of her breasts changes, it may be because of the pregnancy and not the breastfeeding.

Breastfeeding is very convenient to the mother at home or elsewhere. No bottles are required to be washed, sterilized or the feeds prepared. While she is out, she needs only her baby and a clean nappy to go anywhere. A breast fed baby is quieter and happier than a bottle fed baby.

Considering the cost of dried milk, bottles, sterilization, gas or electricity to boil milk and equipment involved in breastfeeding the mother needs only the extra food to eat so as to produce sufficient milk for the baby. In any case, the cost of extra food is lower than the cost of bottle feeding a baby.

Breastfeeding gives you as the mother the advantage

of birth control. You are less likely to conceive during the lactation period. In contrast, the bottle feeding mother is advised to use any form of birth control as soon as she starts having intercourse again.

Breastfeding protects you from eventual likelihood of getting cancer of the breast. Breast cancer is very rare indeed among women who breast feed their babies.

It has been scientifically proved that a breast fed baby is more attached to the mother. Closer relationship seems likely because the baby depends on you only for food. You as the mother are also likely to feed your baby to comfort it instead of just holding it. Studies show that breast fed babies spend more time with their mothers than bottle fed ones.

You are likely to kiss, rock and touch your baby while the bottle fed baby gets a rub, pat and jiggle from her mother. So much are the advantages of your brestfeeding to you and your baby.

All babies should be breastfed exclusively for six months of age and the brestfeeding must be continued till two years or beyond if possible. Before the baby is born, he is protected within your womb against all infections and the protection process is taken over by breastfeeding.

You can successfully breastfeed your baby: that is the most natural way to feed babies. No other milk, food, drink or even water is required. You should breastfeed immediately within one hour of birth. You have to do so unrestrictedly and on demand. Nothing is to be given before the first breastfeed. You can breastfeed even during sickness. No problem for you or the baby.

Breastfeeding reduces post-delivery chances of anaemia. It has a contraceptive effect and also protects against breast as well as ovarian cancers. Obesity is not common among breastfeeding mothers because it helps the mother regain her normal figure. Breastfeeding helps reducing the absenteeism of mothers from work because exclusively breastfed children are less prone to diseases.

Essence: Research shows that the breast fed babies walk earlier than bottle fed babies.

Dos

(1) Continue the exclusive breastfeeding for six months.

(2) Keep on kissing and touching your baby.

Dont's

(1) Have any tension that the shape of your breasts changes because of breastfeeding. It may be because of the pregnancy.

(2) Think that the lactation period is a 100% safe contraceptive.

4

ONSET OF BREAST MILK

Immediately after your baby is born, your breasts start getting full-fledged supply of milk for breastfeeding. While usually many mothers have problems with supplying the right amount of milk, others find inadequate supply of breast milk especially in the early weeks. Too much of milk is often a nuisance for mothers. On the other hand, too little milk, becomes an excuse for some mothers for stopping breastfeeding.

It has been seen that women who really want to breast feed produce more milk than those who don't intend to breast feed or are reluctant to do it. In fact, most women want to breastfeed but fail because they believe that they do not have sufficient milk.

Modern women have normally this excuse. Actually all women can breast feed if they are well prepared and encouraged. Fifty percent of women developed breast milk after they were given oxytoncin injections. This milk otherwise was blocked in the breast and was not available for the baby. Milk supply can always be increased. Only women should know the way of doing so.

You have to see whether your baby is getting enough milk and accordingly should be your milk supply. If the baby is alert, then his consumption would be more. Even if your baby consistently is lagging, yet is well and cheerful; no need to worry. It is not that weight gain indicates how healthy your baby is.

Factors responsible for milk supply

(1) Age of mother—Older mothers having their first babies produce less milk than younger ones. This usually applies to women of more than thirty years of age. However, their milk supply can always be increased.

(2) Attitude of mother—Mothers who really want to breast feed produce more milk. Talking about the attitude of mothers, they preferred to bottle feed giving an excuse that their babies refused the breast. Similarly, mothers who wanted to breastfeed said that their babies refused the bottle. Breastfeeding is thus greatly helped by positive attitudes.

(3) Suckling—The more you suckle your baby, the more prolactin is secreted by the pituitary gland and more milk is produced by your breasts. Total suckling time is important and that depends on the number and length of the feeds. You should always give a certain number of feeds your baby asks for. Sometimes, you have to offer your baby unasked for feeds to build up your milk supply.

(4) Degree of emptying the breast— If your baby is not allowed to empty the breast or if the breast is allowed to remain full for a long period before the baby gets feeds then the milk supply will gradually go down. Hence, whenever you feel your breasts full or uncomfortable, you should give your baby a feed.

(5) Diet—You should eat slightly more food of better quality and drink according to your thirst so as to produce the required quality of milk for your baby.

(6) Be calm and never be in a hurry.

Don't do anything in a hurry. Maintain calmness and cut out the things which worry you. Relax both before and during feeds. It all comes through practice. Cut down on other activities so that you have enough time for the feeds.

(7) Meet the demands of your baby - If your baby has been previously well satisfied with your feed but suddenly starts feeling hungry after a feed, then you must increase your milk supply to meet his demands, give him some extra feeds during the day. Increased nipple stimulation will soon increase your milk production. Your milk supply would depend upon the frequency of breast feeding your baby.

Essence: Age, attitude and diet of mother besides art of feeding the baby are solely responsible for production of adequate breast milk.

Dos

(1) Eat more of quality food and take fluids to produce the necessary milk for your baby

(2) Give frequent feeds to your baby to keep your milk supply intact.

Don'ts

(1) Do anything in a hurry. Take it easy before and during the feed.

(2) Get frustrated if by chance, enough milk is not produced by you.

•••5•••

GENERATION OF BREAST MILK

With the onset of a girl's periods, changes in the shape and size of her breasts and nipples carry on until her late teens. They remain the same till she becomes pregnant.

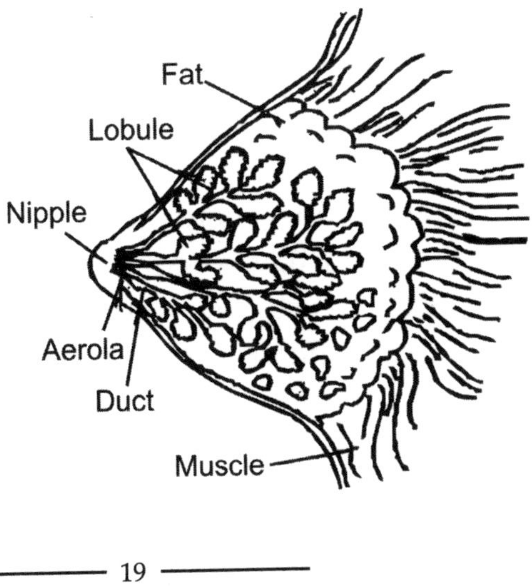

Your breasts are made up of various small segments each containing glandular tissue leading to a main duct opening at the nipple. The milk flows out of the breast through nipple pores or holes at the end of your nipples. When your baby gets attached to your breast, the mouth of the baby opens wide enough to take as much breast as possible. This would stimulate the nerves of your brain for the hormones of milk-making, prolactin and milk flow, oxytocin to come back to your breast via your blood supply.

In case your baby does not have enough after of the breast in the mouth to stimulate the nerves around the areolathe darker skin around your nipple, less hormone will be released with the result you will not produce as much milk as you need to because of the low prolactin level, baby gets less milk due to low oxytocin level and you feel pain in your nipples since baby will be chewing the nipple instead of breastfeeding. Obviously, your baby wants a feed almost constantly to get enough food.

Your breasts during pregnancy

With the onset of your first period, you had some breast growth with production of hormones estrogen and progesterone. Thereafter, a small amount of breast growth would have occurred during each menstrual cycle. Such breast growth continues during each cycle until around the age of thirty. During pregnancy the breasts go through three main phases to prepare for breastfeeding

Phase I - Appearance of milk line

The embryo has a milk line from the armpit to the groin by the sixth week of its development. The growth continues in the breast tissue and the nipples tend to migrate to the usual place on the chest anywhere along this line. Normally, women have extra breast tissue in their armpits that fills up with milk when the milk comes in during the first week.

Phase II - Hormone changes for breast development

There are apparent changes in your breasts as and when you missed a period which is the initial sign of pregnancy during which many hormones are involved in growth of milk making sacs and the ducts. Prolactin is important in the growth of the breasts but does not help to make milk during pregnancy. You would observe that there will be a small amount of colostrum in your breasts from twelve weeks

Phase III - When the baby is born

As you deliver the baby, the main breastfeeding hormone, prolactin, prevailing in your bloodstream is now able to start the milk-making process. Every time baby sucks, more prolactin is released and so your milk supply builds up.

Oxytocin, a hormone of love, labour and lactation is also released into the bloodstream when you first start thinking about whether the baby needs a feed. This hormone flows through your body during orgasm bringing wonderful feelings of tenderness towards your partner.

A huge amount of oxytocin is released and it is that which acts on muscles of your uterus and causes them to contract and push your baby out. It also gives you a wonderful feeling of affection towards your baby and you would like to caress it.

Quantity of milk produced by your breasts

How much milk your breasts make depends upon the following factors.

Size of breast - Small or large breasts work in the same way. It is not necessary that the breasts of bigger size produce more milk. Your breasts would produce the milk as it is taken out of them irrespective of whether you are feeding one baby or more.

Reduced breast growth - Even if size of your breasts does not change during pregnancy, it does not mean that you will make less milk. You may take the advice of the doctor to increase the hormones you are taking to assist breast growth during pregnancy and milk-making after your baby is born.

Breast surgery - Women often go in for breast surgery which may be for the removal of a breast lump, a breast reduction or for breast implants. In all the cases, surgery is conducted in such a way that it does not come in your way of breastfeeding. Exceptionally there may be some complications which can be looked into accordingly so that your breastfeeding can be restored to be normal. If you have had breast surgery, make an appointment with the lactation consultant and also be in touch with breastfeeding support group for information and necessary guidance. All these have a vital role in production of breast milk

Essence: Size of your breasts doesn't matter. Small or large breasts do produce the adequate quantity needed by your baby.

Dos

1) Take care that your baby has enough portion of your breast including areola, the dark skin around your nipple in its month.
2) Extend your affection towards your baby.

Don'ts

1) Have an impression that you will make less milk because the size of your breasts did not change during pregnancy
2) Hesitate to consult the specialist if you had earlier any surgical problem in your breasts.

…6…

LEARNING TO BREASTFEED

If you happen to see videos of babies an hour after birth you would come to know how the babies move their heads and elbows backward and forward to arrive at the nipple. When the baby is comfortable with the feed then the mother too develops affection and tenderness towards the baby. Thereafter, you enjoy the breastfeeding and become used to it.

Know your breasts

Even during pregnancy, you should know about your breasts. You usually wash them once and dry them but during breastfeeding you have to do that frequently. Before the baby is born you should give a gentle massage bringing your thumb as well as fingers towards your areolas and nipples. As a result you may find a drop or two of colostrum.

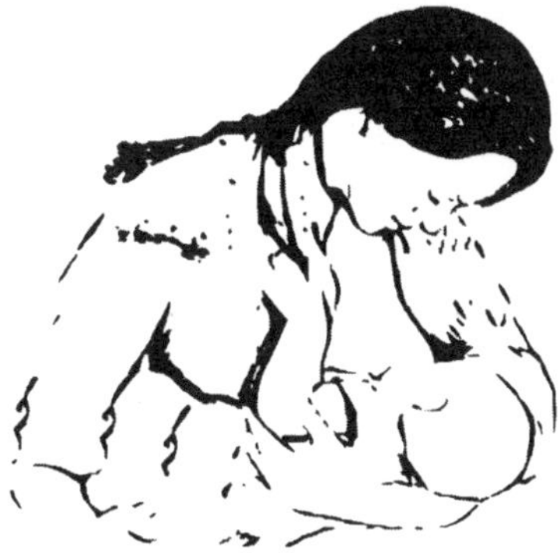

Find a comfortable position that works well for you.

The bottom gums of newly born babies are a little behind their top gums. The same are to be positioned so that their chin is lifted up and accordingly pushed gently into a mother's breast so as to bring their bottom jaw and tongue forward. In order to make it comfortable for your baby also you will need to have a grip on the tip of your nipple.

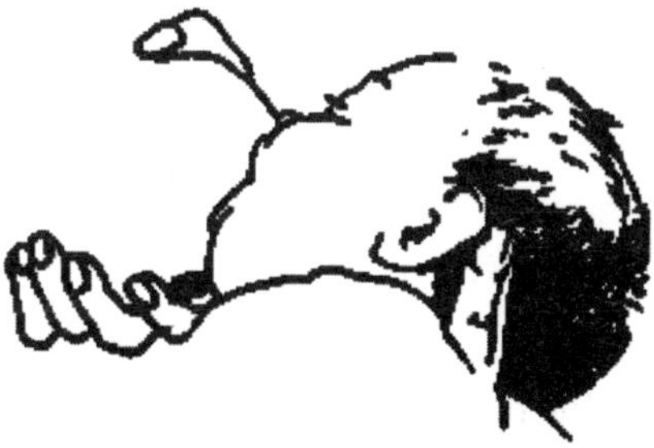

Hold the breast in your hand with thumb on top and fingers below the breast. Place the baby on your breast and see:

1. Is baby's mouth widely opened
2. Are baby's lips curled out
3. Is baby's chin touching your breast.

See that when the baby's tongue is flat it will draw milk from your breast by a rolling motion from the front to back of the tongue. Practise the way you find yourself in the most comfortable position and attach your baby to your bosom. Try both the poses of sitting up and lying down. You would certainly love and enjoy breastfeeding.

To make breastfeeding interesting and attractive for baby point your nipple to the nose of the baby, rub the lower side of your areola on his bottom lip with your nipple above his top lip. When his mouth is wide open and his tongue is forward over his bottom gum, immediately bring him towards you. Relax and enjoy feeding him.

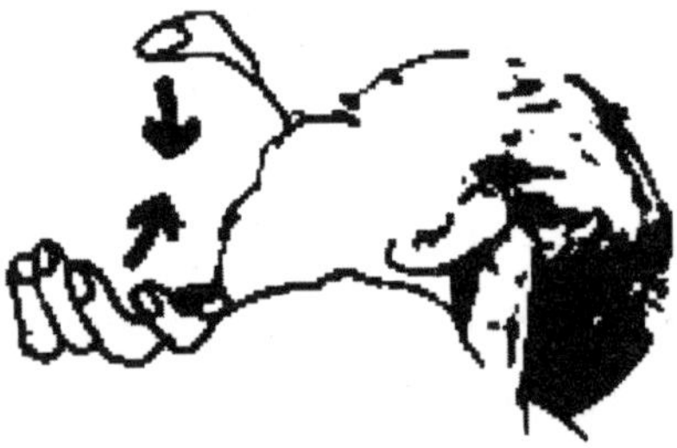

In case baby falls asleep squeeze your breast gently to help your milk flow. This will make your baby start sucking again.

Learning by hand

During pregnancy itself, you can express a drop or two of milk onto your nipple to smell and lick. This course of action you can do by placing your thumb on the edge of areola and fingers on its opposite side. Push your thumb and fingers towards each other through the breast until you feel them touch. Relax and continue the slow squeeze and repeat steps eight to ten times. If you are able to perform it easily every day then you would find that a drop of milk will appear on your nipple. This is how you learn by hand.

Essence: It is interesting to see how the new born babies immediately after birth move their heads and elbows to arrive at the nipple.

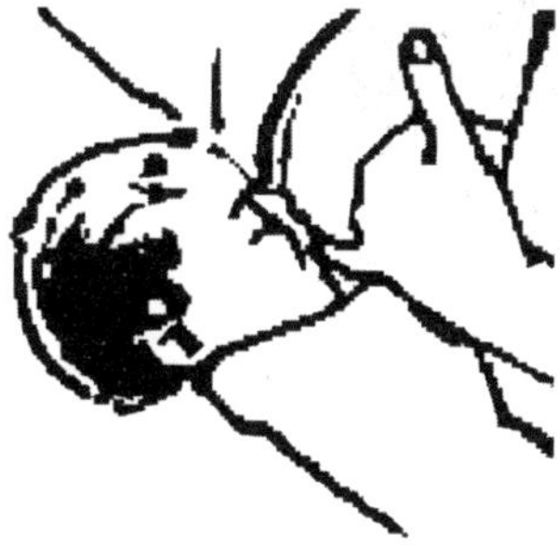

If you want to take the baby off your breast, slip your finger in between baby's mouth and gums to break the suction.

Dos

(1) Learn about breastfeeding during your pregnancy itself

(2) Try to breasfeed your baby in sitting up as well as lying down positions.

Don'ts

(1) Start breastfeeding without any proper guidance

(2) Be away from your baby for a longer duration, once the breastfeed has commenced.

•••7•••

HOW DO INFANTS RECOGNISE THEIR MOM?

A baby crying stops doing so when mother takes him in her lap. It is interesting to note that the infants use all their senses such as sight, smell, taste, touch and hearing to recognise their mom so as to continue breastfeeding.

Babies are quite intelligent and start scanning the faces of mother and father the moment they look at them. Babies need to be less than 20 centimetres away from your face to see you well.

Small raised pimple like areas on your areola so called montgomery follicles produce a substance called sebum that not only lubricates your nipple and areola but has an enticing smell. Besides, babies are able to recognise you with the smell of your milk and body.

Your baby knows the taste of your breast milk as he licks the colostrum from your areola and nipple. Baby takes out the tongue when he enjoys the breastfeeding.

You are recognised by your baby for the softness of your body and the warmth it radiates. Your baby also knows you by your heartbeats which he has been listening to right from pregnancy. Baby is also very well aware of the sound pitch of your talking.

Baby needs calmness without any loud noise to listen to your voice and sounds. This is how your baby feeds all programmes in his brain which works as a computer for him enabling him to recognise you with the above mentioned senses.

Essence: Your baby recognises you through his senses like sight, smell, taste, touch and hearing your voice.

Dos

(1) Talk to your baby politely and softly

(2) Be in touch with your baby constantly as it enhances the emotional bond with him.

Don'ts

1) Shout or make loud noise in presence of your baby as he needs calmness

2) Think that your baby doesn't know anything. He feeds all programmes in his brain

•••8•••

PREPARING FOR BREASTFEEDING

Before giving birth to baby, during the antenatal period, you can discuss about breastfeeding with your health care provider. You can also talk to your husband and elders of your family on the topic because during exclusive breastfeeding, you would be needing their co-operation. You have to interact specifically with a mother who has recently breastfed her own baby. She will be able to reply to your many questions and would also guide you to better things. Take full advantage of such a mother.

Throughout your pregnancy and breastfeeding, you need to eat a balanced diet from all food groups covering energy giving food in the form of cereals, starchy roots, tubers, sugar, nuts, fats and oils besides body building food which includes milk and milk products, eggs, meat, fish, pulses, legumes, nuts, oil seeds, green vegetables and fruits. You have to take extra food during pregnancy so as to meet additional requirements. Alcohol and smoking are to be avoided during pregnancy. While you are pregnant, take care of your nipples and breasts. Don't apply any special soap or oil.

To optimise the benefits of breastfeeding, you have to breastfeed your baby continuously for the first six months. As soon as your baby is born, you have to initiate the breastfeeding preferably within an hour of birth. At this time, the new born is very active after which he goes to sleep. In case of caesarian delivery, your baby may start suckling within three to four hours or as soon the effect of anaesthesia is over.

To start breastfeeding immediately after birth, hold the baby close to your breast for skin touch contact. Baby will open his mouth widely as you touch him around his mouth. Offer him the whole breast at this time and he would gladly take a mouthful of the breast. Milk flow is stimulated through skin-to-skin contact thereby helping to strengthen better mother-child bonding and development of baby.

Please ensure that only your breast milk is baby's first food. So as to establish successive breastfeeding, no foods such as sugar, water, any other milk food or drink should be given. In fact, such feeds retard the production and supply of breast milk, create nipple confusion and increase risk of infection.

On demand feed your baby till he is satisfied. When he gets satisfaction, he himself will release the nipple. You may offer alternate breasts at each feed. This way your baby receives both fore milk and hind milk.

You should establish good and correct breastfeeding skills that help in an effective milk transfer from you to the baby. You can feed your baby lying down or in a sitting position which is comfortable to you. Baby must have free access to the breast. It is to be taken care of because poor positioning often results in poor attachment.

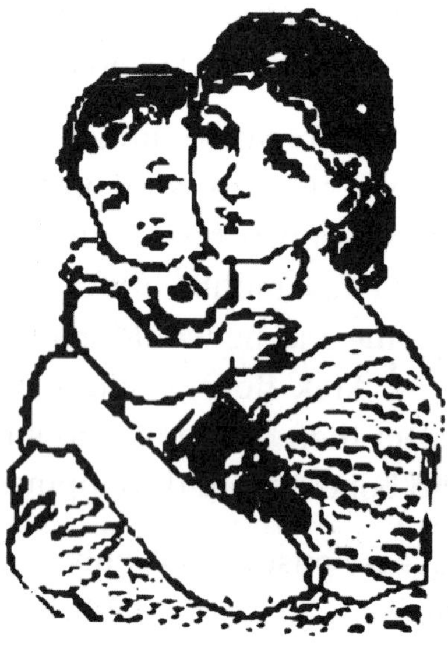

For feeding, the right position is not that your baby should have his head straight with you holding him. He should face the breast with his nose opposite to your nipple and also his body close to you. You have to support baby's entire body, not just the neck and shoulder.

Your nipple has to touch the infant's mouth, as he opens his mouth widely. Offer the whole breast to him to get as much as he can into his mouth.

Please note that in a good position for feeding the baby should have his neck straight or bent slightly back. His body tilted towards you as well as close to you and well supported. There has to be eye contact between you and your baby. Failing all these are recognized as poor positioning.

Apart from closeness, comfort and pleasure, babies must suckle effectively, your baby must take enough of the breast in his mouth. A good attachment includes clean touching breast, mouth wide open, lower lip turned outward besides more of areola visible above than below the mouth without any sign of pain.

In case your baby is not well attached it may result in pain and damage your nipple due to ineffective removal of breast milk. While in effective suckling, you can notice that baby suckles with few deep sucks. Sometimes you find he pauses and you see or hear the infant swallowing the milk.

Coming to duration of suckling the pattern varies with some babies fulfilling their needs in about ten minutes while others take longer feeds. There seems to be some problem if the baby takes feed for a very short time say about five minutes or if he takes longer feeds for more than an hour. In low birth-weight-babies, breastfeeds may be long which is considered as normal.

You must feed your baby on demand with at least more than eight feeds in 24 hours. Initially the frequency is more but later it reduces. You have to feed baby as frequently and as long as he wants to round the clock. Breastfeeding at night helps maintain the milk supply as more prolactin is secreted at that time. Satisfied child releases breast spontaneously and the mothers do not have to stop breastfeeding.

You have to feed your baby from one breast completely and after that only put the baby on the second breast. This way both the breasts get equal stimulation for milk production.

Essence: To prepare for breastfeeding, you have to interact specifically with a mother who has recently breast fed her own baby

Dos

Ensure that only your breast milk is baby's best food.

Don'ts

Feed your baby from one breast only, keep on interchanging the breast and this way both the breasts get equal stimulation for milk production.

...9...

TOUCH THERAPY FOR MOTHER AND CHILD

It has been seen that your baby does not gain much weight so long as you are in the hospital and your baby is in an incubator. Baby starts gaining weight as soon as he is taken out from the incubator and transferred to your lap. Here the conventional touch therapy takes place between you and your baby. You would find that your baby becomes fit, fine and active when he comes in close contact with you. This touch therapy can occur for varying periods depending upon your baby's health and needs to occur daily. This touch therapy resembles the famous Australian kangaroo mother care.

As part of touch therapy, the babies are dressed in

nappies and when they have skin touch with father or especially mother. Then their mothers can alter their own temperature to increase or lower their baby's temperature besides developing higher levels of oxygen in their blood, babies cry less, gain weight quickly and they are breastfed for a longer period.

By virtue of touch therapy, you produce more of breast milk and your baby is less likely to have an abnormally slow heart rate or suffer from long pauses between breaths. These positive outcomes occur if the said therapy works for about half an hour every day and even babies assisted by a ventilator for their breathing get these benefits.

Your baby would always look warm and comfortable on your chest apart from the fact that you and your baby are going to develop sensitive and long lasting tenderness of love and affection with the help of this touch therapy.

Essence: The touch therapy works as a miracle that superbly bonds you with your baby.

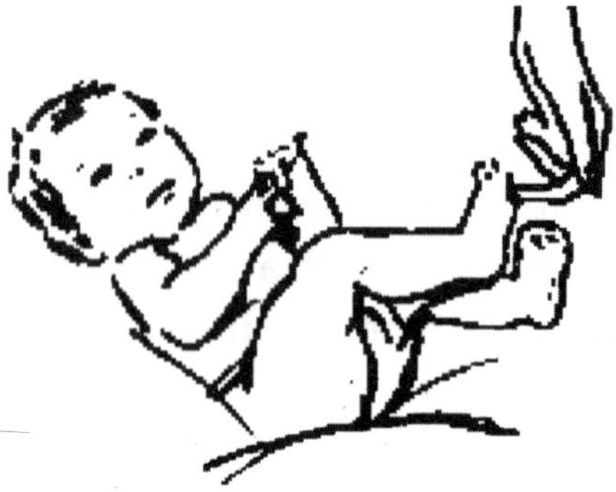

Dos

Try to maintain

your skin-to-skin contact with your baby as soon as he is born and thereafter continue to do so consistently.

Don'ts

Get panicky if due to some reason you have to be away from your baby for a long time.

··10··

KNOWING YOUR BABY

During breastfeeding so called lactation period, the mother feeds the baby regularly. Accordingly, mom needs to know the behaviour of babies. They should be able to judge the requirement of babies when they weep or cry. Going back to grandmother's child health bulletin which states that the mother has to feed her baby five times a day apart from a fixed bath time, sun bath time and play time for an hour and a half each day; the rest of the day was for sleep. But babies don't go by the bulletin or chart of grandmas. Their demand is erratic in the entire cycle of day and night.

Mother has to feed her baby a low protein milk eight to twelve times a day so as to double the weight of baby in three months. Mother's milk assists in optimal

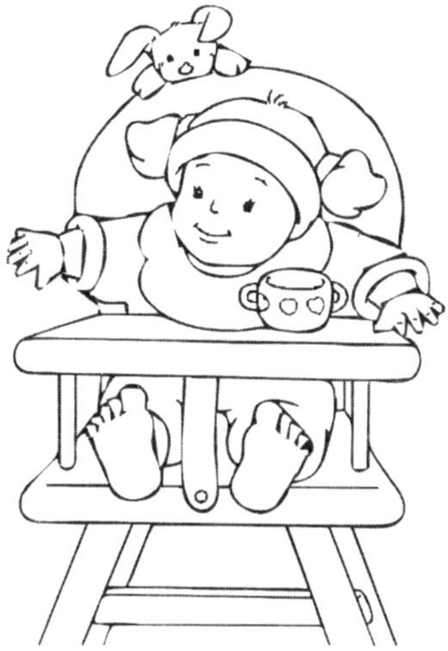

growth of the brain and spinal cord of baby because of the presence of fatty acids in human milk. These are converted to longer chain polyunsaturated fatty acids needed for nervous system, sharpness and acuteness of sight.

Nearly half the calories in human milk are provided by carbohydrates specifically lactose that helps the infant to absorb iron and calcium. The lactobacillus combines with another factor in human milk which in turn leads to high levels of lactic acid in the baby's intestines to stop the growth of harmful bacteria. Human milk is low in protein and it is broken down in the baby's stomach very quickly. Mother's milk in the form of breastfeeding is an amazing food for babies

Essence: Mother's milk enhances development of brain and spinal cord of baby

Dos

1) Try to know the needs of your baby when he weeps or cries
2) Watch minutely the demands of feeds of baby during day time and night.

Don'ts

1) Go by grandma's chart of feeding
2) Think that baby needs only feed when he cries. He may have some other problem for which medication is required.

••11••

SOLUTIONS OF BREAST FEEDING PROBLEMS

Breastfeeding is a` unique and cherishable natural experience for every mother. You often come across some problems which may result in discontinuation of breastfeeding or providing certain alternative supplements to the baby. Problems include flat, inverted, sore nipples, engorgement of breasts, swelling or insufficient milk. Such problems can be prevented if you take proper care to prepare your breastfeeding right from pregnancy. A few of these problems pertain to shape and size of nipple besides breast tissue.

Nipple Protractility

Gently pull out your nipples which if they stand errect are working for breastfeeding. This is so called Nipple Protractility. The length of nipple doesn't matter and don't worry about flat nipples. The nipple just guides the baby where he has to take the breast.

An inverted nipple doesn't become erect and when you pull it out, rather it goes deeper into the breast. Actually inverted nipples are very rarely seen and usually nipples become normal during pregnancy itself.

Sometimes baby sucks your nipple only which makes your nipple long. So bring the baby closer to the breast to enable him to catch more of breast tissue into his mouth. If the feeding continues in poor or incorrect position, it may lead to sore and cracked nipples.

In case you feel pain during breastfeeding, you must wait till your baby finishes his feed. Bring your baby in correct position and your pain will go. Continue the breastfeeding on the affected breast because sore nipples normally heal when the suckling position is corrected.

Cracked nipples can be treated by feeding in correct position, washing the nipples daily once only with water and exposing the nipples to air and sun to the maximum possible. You may also put a drop of your hind milk on the nipple after each feed and it would help you in your painless breastfeeding. Avoid medicated creams which may increase the soreness.

Another common problem is the fullness and engorgement of breasts. Milk keeps on coming continuously and if it is not drained then engorgement of breasts may occur. The engorged breasts are tight and very painful. Delayed starting of breastfeeds and early detachment of baby from the breast are among the common causes of engorged breasts.

Your baby is unable to take feed properly from the engorged breast because of poor attachment. It leads to inadequate emptying. Breast engorgement is prevented by avoiding other feeds given before breastfeeding, keeping constant touch of baby with mother, feeding in right position, unrestricted and exclusive breastfeeding on demand.

Sometimes it so happens that the baby doesn't suckle well on a particular segment of the breast, with the result the thick milk blocks the milk duct which causes painful hard swelling. This problem can be treated by feeding the baby frequently on the affected breast in different suckling positions for quick emptying of the breasts, massaging the lump towards the nipple or by taking rest and wearing loose clothes.

The breast becomes red, hot and swollen and it is called mastitis if the blockage of duct persists or engorgement remains. As a part of its treatment, express the milk frequently and continue breastfeeding, alleviating pain with warm water fomentation, draining the affected breast as soon as possible.

You find leakage of milk from the breast during the first few weeks of lactation. It usually happens at the time of feed or when you have affectionate thoughts about your baby. Take it easy, it is all normal

Many nursing mothers find a little blood in their milk though there is no nipple fissure. You can continue breastfeeding as it is usually a harmless and self-limiting condition.

Essence: Common problems during breastfeeding are related to nipples, swelling of breasts and insufficient milk supply

Dos

1) Take care of problems pertaining to shape and size of nipples besides breast tissue right from pregnancy
2) Feed your baby in correct position and pain of your nipples will go

Don'ts

1) Wash your nipples every now and then
2) Apply medicated creams on nipples

··12··

BREAST FEEDING AND LIFE STYLE CHANGES

When you are breastfeeding your little baby, you have to do it around ten times throughout 24 hours. Each feed normally takes about an hour. So about 10 to 12 hours your baby keeps you busy in breastfeeding thereby changing your lifestyle. This consumption of time by baby is exclusive of extra washing, drying and folding of clothes.

New born babies usually do not sleep in the evenings from say 5pm to 10 pm. During this period, you ought to keep the baby occupied with toys or some other way. So the prime time of your evening entertaiment is gone.

With breastfeeding you become unfashionable

because now-a-days most mothers are bottle feeding their babies as they don't have time to breastfeed. Earlier only wealthy persons could afford to buy milk powder but gradually this concept is spreading through all the social groups and the middle classes are leading the way of bottle feeding.

Many women feel that breastfeeding makes them less sexy for themselves and their husbands. Due to the cult of the breast as a sex object the speed of breastfeeding has certainly declined. Perhaps the present trend among young women doing so without bras attracts the male.

Breasts in our society have been equated with sex and obviously run the risk of people turning to stare at them. You always feel this fear of embarrassment. Though TV and other areas of the media start showing mothers feeding their babies still acceptability by women tends to be slow.

No doubt, you feel hurt because when you breastfeed you have sore nipples and sometimes you have other painful breast conditions. Of course, soreness of nipples is temporary, easily curable and avoidable.

Moreover, breastfeeding is inconvenient for you as it ties you with your baby. You have to be attached with your baby for at least four to six months constantly. In the first few weeks, you have to limit your outings because your baby won't remain for long without feeds.

You don't know the quantity of breast milk consumed by your baby because God has not made the breast transparent. So your baby would stick to your breast till he is satisfied. During breastfeeding if the baby starts crying it means that your breast milk supply is inadequate.

Since you have to feed your baby more often, your household work will suffer especially if you have other children too. You have to co-relate your feeds with your baby in such a way that the night feeds do not interfere with your sleep.

In remote cases, sometimes you get fear that you will fail in breastfeeding and as a result, it often happens so. This produces long lasting psychological impact coupled with a deep sense of disappointment. You have maintained your balance of mind and see that the fear should not dare to penetrate your body. You always get encouragement from nurses, doctors and your senior family members. You should not lose heart and keep on doing the things as per their guidance. Accordingly, you would be a successful and proud breastfeeding mother.

Essence: New born babies normally do not sleep during your prime time of social and entertainment period from 5 pm to 10 pm.

Dos

3) Limit your outings for the first few weeks as your baby won't be long without feeds.

4) Co-relate your feeds with your baby so that your night sleep is not disturbed.

Don'ts

3) Take breastfeeding as unfashionable, you have to look after the health of your baby

4) Feel that breastfeeding in public is sexual embarrassment.

13

ENGORGEMENT OF BREASTS

As you know your baby has been getting sufficient food in the form of your wonderful amniotic fluid right from the twelfth week of your pregnancy apart from lovely brown fat your baby has acquired around the neck and shoulders during the last few weeks of pregnancy. With the result your baby does not need your milk at least for 48 hours. So to say, your breasts would be loaded fully with milk but your baby initially won't be consuming your milk. Obviously, milk would start leaking from both your breasts.

To avoid this engorgement of your breasts, let your baby suck one breast. When the baby gets satisfied, detach him from one breast and put him on your other breast. Thus, this equal drainage over the day and suckling for long periods prevents your breasts from becoming engorged when your milk pours in.

As the second day after your delivery passes, your breasts are able to make a lot of milk showing many veins on your chest and breasts. Blood supply occurs due to this change causing some swelling in the tissue of the breasts resulting in venous engorgement. It all happens as the arteries are bringing a lot of blood to your breasts whereas the veins are taking it away very slowly.

The easiest way to overcome breast engorgement is to put something cold on your breasts. This effect of coolness would tighten the blood vessels and gradually the swelling would subside over the next 48 hours.

Some women suffer from milk engorgement which occurs if the breasts have not been well drained or may be excess amount of hormone prolactin has been produced by the mother.

For relieving this milk engorgement of breasts, you have to feed your baby alternatively from each of your breasts and after each feed you have to apply cold packs to both your breasts.

Some babies have a chance of getting milk in large quantities. Baby has by the time learnt a good suck-swallow on-breathe sequence but if the flow is so fast then baby will need to be positioned accordingly to cope with it. What you need to do is to tilt his head so that he can gulp the milk quickly. Your baby should have the demand for your milk supply available.

Essence: Your breasts would get hot and hard making you uneasy if the same are not drained out in time.

Dos

1) Keep on feeding your baby with switch over from one breast to the other at frequent intervals
2) Express your milk if baby is not able to consume that much intake.

Don'ts

1) Take bath with water because it will expand blood vessels and increase the swelling
2) Apply any cream or lotion on your breasts which may worsen the problem.

··14··

NIPPLE SORENESS AND PAIN

It is a common problem faced by many breastfeeding mothers when they experience pain in their nipples in the beginning of breastfeeding particularly in the first week. Such problems affect 10 to 80 per cent of breastfeeding mothers. Of course, it is not possible to prevent the nipple becoming painful but the situation can be prevented to make the condition from getting worse.

The main cause of nipple pain is the position of holding the baby which makes it difficult to attach your baby to your breast so as to suck and swallow your milk without squashing your nipple. After the baby is born, your milk flow becomes fast in the initial three or four days. Your baby will try to gulp every mouthful. If the chin of the baby is not lifted up into your breast, your baby would squash your nipple against the roof of his mouth which causes the pain to your nipples.

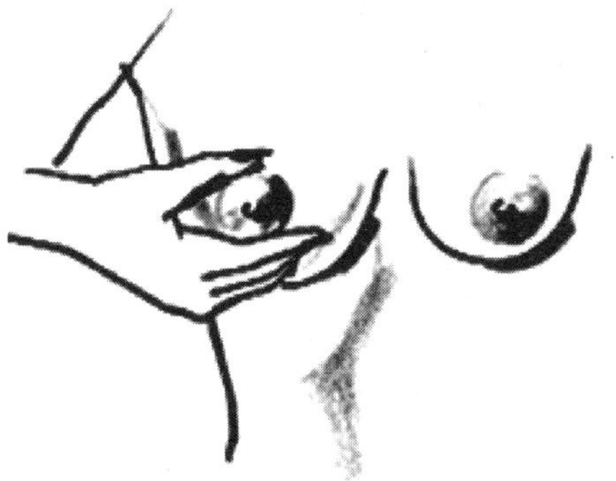

Express some breast milk on the nipples and the dark area around after feeding your baby. Put up your bra after that milk gets dry.

The pain of sore nipples begins with the breastfeeding for a minute or two but not throughout the feed. Peak of nipple soreness occurs on the third day and by the fourth day, it is reducing. Babies fed on four-hourly schedule may damage the nipple skin as they suck more being so hungry.

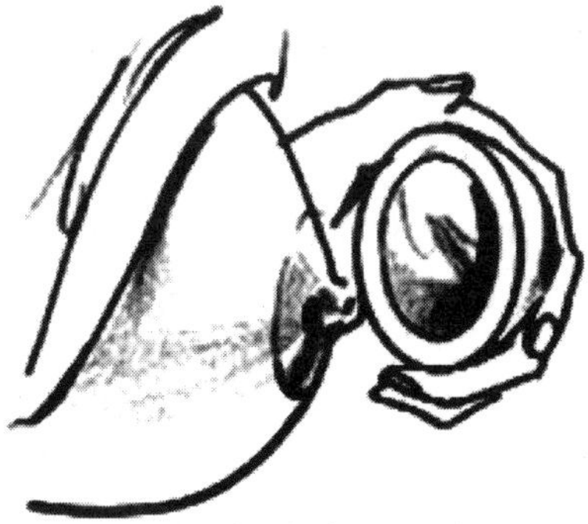

You may also wear a breast shell under your bra to help protect the sore nipples from rubbing against your bra.

You should always find a right person who can rightly diagnose the soreness of your nipples and give you the proper guidance to make breastfeeding comfortable and enjoyable.

Sometimes, your nipples are painful because of your baby's sucking. Your friends and relatives may advise you that sore nipples get better gradually which may discourage you from seeking help.

Undermentioned are a few guidelines to treat your sore nipples, the cardinal rule being to carry on feeding without stopping.

Importantly, make sure that your baby is positioned well at the breast. Sit up or you can even lean slightly forward in such a way that your baby is not tugging at the nipple but is well supported. The baby should have a part or the full areola in his mouth and not just the nipple. Change the position of your feeding during the day which would ensure that no single part of your nipple is painfully affected.

Feed your baby on demand only. Don't limit drinking time but limit total suckling time. Suckling to comfort your baby while he sleeps after he has finished drinking is good practice when your nipples are not sore. It will also help you in healing if you take him off the breast at this very stage in the first week or so if you have sore nipples.

Don't soak your nipples in bath water as the moisture makes soreness last longer. Always offer the less sore nipple first. Take an aspirin a short time before a feed if you feel that the pain in your nipples is inhibiting.

Carefully, expose your damaged nipple skin to sun

failing which you can try exposing your nipples to light from an electric light bulb. Don't remove any crusts which appear on the nipples. It is a healing process.

Moreover, try to expose your nipples to the air as much as possible. You can sleep without a bra at night and allow the air to circulate under your top clothes. Wear your bra as soon as the soreness has healed up. Air helps tremendously.

Normally after the fifth day, a few women develop a crack or a fissure in the nipples. It develops at the base of the nipple and is acutely painful needing prompt treatment. If the fissure doesn't heal within a few days, you may have to take the baby off the breast. Some mothers can continue to feed with the use of a nipple shield in which case intensive care must be taken to keep it clean.

There are various reasons why you develop soreness and pain in your nipples while breastfeeding which is the usual problem many women come across in the first week in particular. But every problem has a solution. At the same time there are several ways to overcome the problem to continue to completely drain your breasts while feeding.

Essence: Expose your sore painful nipples to the air as much as possible

Dos

1) Feed your baby in a properly directed position
2) Be careful for the first three days of feeding as peak of soreness occurs on the third day and gets reduced from the fourth day.

Don'ts

1) Soak your nipples in bath water as the moiture makes soreness last longer
2) Wear bra at night if you have soreness of nipples. Allow the air to circulate under your top clothes

··15··

CAESARIAN SECTION AND BREAST FEEDING

Normally a caesarian delivery should not affect breastfeeding. During the operation, depending upon the health of the mother an injection of anesthesia is given to her and there may be some effect of it on baby as well.

In spite of anaesthetic feeling you should be in a position to breastfeed within the first hour after the birth of your baby. You should also go for touch therapy which may not be allowed in hospital but you should always request the hospital authorities for the skin-to-skin touch therapy. It is very much possible in private nursing homes.

Usually many women are told that their breast milk

would come later incase of a caesarian delivery. But what actually needs to happen for milk production to commence is for the placenta to be delivered and your nipples to be stimulated. Placenta will be delivered by the doctor as a part of the operation whereas skin-to-skin therapy is necessary for nipple stimulation by virtue of which the milk comes to your breasts.

Now the milk has arrived in your breast after which you have to take care of your milk supply. The baby should get the feeds as per the prescribed schedule. You have to see that your post-operative stitches are not affected while you breast feed your baby.

Often, mothers are advised to rest their babies on a pillow under their arm so called the twin position putting babies, feet behind them which lessens the weight over the operation site in the early days. However, there are numerous positions to sit or lie down to feed your baby. The same are very useful in case of a caesarian section.

Essence: Most women across the world having undergone caesarian section have been able to breastfeed their babies exclusively with little assistance

Dos

1) Try to maintain skin-to-skin touch therapy with your baby for which make request to hospital

authorities even in case of caesarian section.

Don'ts

1) Lose your confidence and you will be in a position to breast feed your baby successfully in spite of the surgical operation.

··16··

HORMONAL CHANGES

During your lactation period, the level of your hormones normally affects your sexual interest. Some women claim that they are less easily aroused while others say that their libido is heightened. Most nursing mothers suffer from sleep deprivation with sex being the last thing on their minds.

There are various hormones such as oestrogen, oxytocin and gonadotropin releasing hormones to control your sexuality and fertility while you are breastfeeding.

After your delivery, your oestrogen levels will be low until just before your first ovulation. This hormone keeps your vagina lubricated making you feel more sexy. So the low levels may affect your libido.

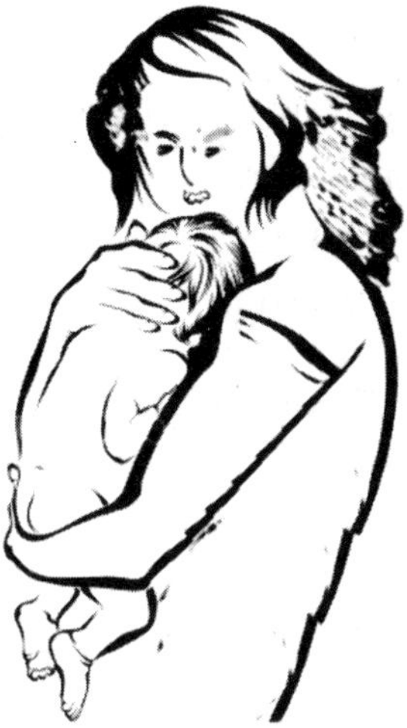

Oxytocin is released by virtue of love, labour and lactation making you feel good. During sexual intercourse, oxytocin is released and your breasts will leak. Hence feed the baby first and keep a towel in bed to catch the flow. Breast milk is good for your partner as well as your baby. Enjoy knowing that there will by plenty of milk in your breast for your baby too, if he wakes up.

Gonadotropin-releasing hormone so called as GnRH is the hormone that acts to begin ovulation. The suckling continues round the clock and the interest of your baby in suckling is not affected by solids. So GnRH will be kept at a low level and ovulation is less likely to occur. The mechanism that suppresses ovulation is the regular nipple stimulation of breastfeeding. It leads to high levels of endorphins that stop the release of GnRH.

It has been established that breastfeeding in almost 99 per cent cases has been effective as a contraceptive in case your baby is less than six months old or you have not had a menstrual period since the birth of your baby or if your baby is waking for feeds during the night or your baby is not having other drinks/solids or your baby is not frequently suckling on a dummy. You need to use other contraceptive methods in case there is a change in any of the above points.

Please note that use of a dummy can lead to pregnancy. Even if your baby has it for five minutes before or after each feed which way lead to rise in your GnRH level, you may ovulate. So be careful otherwise you will have to adopt another method of contraception. Prevention is better than cure.

Essence: During breastfeeding various hormones are released to control your sexuality and fertility

Dos

1) Oestrogen hormone makes you feel more sexy. You can take advantage of it and enjoy sex with you husband even during breastfeeding.

Don'ts

Be worried that the milk will not be available for your baby if he wakes up while you are offering it to your partner.

··17··

DIFFERENT TERMS OF BREAST MILK

Breast milk is an ideal food containing all the nutrients necessary for baby's initial six months of life. At different stages of lactation, it is defined by different terms namely colostrum, transition milk, mature milk, fore milk, hind milk, preterm milk and term milk.

Colostrum - It is special milk that is thick, sticky and yellowish or clear in colour produced by a woman during the first few days after delivery. It has large quantities of protective substances and growth factors besides containing more proteins as well as vitamins A and K than mature milk.

Development and maturation of the baby's gastrointestinal tract is enhanced by colostrum. It is secreted in small quantities (30 to 90ml) and is sufficient to meet the caloric needs of a normal newborn baby for the initial few days of life.

Colostrum has a mild purgative effect that helps to clear baby's first very dark stool and also prevents jaundice. It stimulates the baby's immature intestines to develop so as to digest and absorb milk as well as to prevent the absorption of undigested protein.

In case a baby is given any other milk or food before colostrum, it can damage the intestine and become a potential cause of allergies. Colostrum feeding provides immune factors besides hospital infections, diarrhoea, pneumonia and nosocomial infections etc.

Transition Milk

Following the colostrum stage during the first two weeks, the milk increases in quantity with changes in appearance and composition. Fat and sugar contents increase while the immunoglobulins and protein contents decrease. The breasts feel full, hard and heavy at this time. It is termed as transition milk.

Mature Milk

Though it appears thinner, it increases in quantity containing all the nutrients required for healthy physical and mental development of the baby. It even changes during the length of a single feed suiting the needs of a baby.

Fore Milk

It is the milk that comes in the beginning of a feed that is called fore milk. It is watery and bluish in colour with a low level of fat and high in sugar, proteins, vitamins as well as minerals. It gives satisfaction to baby's thirst and is produced in larger amounts than hind milk. Mothers are sometimes worried because this milk is very thin at first. But it is important for a baby to have fore milk and hind milk so as to get a complete meal and the water which a baby needs.

Hind Milk

Milk that comes later in a feed with extra fat looking whiter than fore milk is known as hind milk satisfying the baby's hunger and supplies more of energy of a breastfeed. Don't take the baby off the breast quickly. Babies who are fed fore and hind milk sleep well remaining healthy. Baby gains weight with feed of fore milk and hind milk

Preterm Milk

Milk produced by a woman having delivered prematurely is called preterm milk. It has more protein, minerals, immunoglobulins and lactoferrin than mature milk most suitable for needs of preterm baby for survival and growth. It is essential food for low birth weight babies.

Term Milk

Milk produced by women with full term delivery is known as term milk. Composition of milk changes according to the gestational age or the maturity of the baby. So the milk produced by a woman who has full term delivery varies from composition point of view to the milk produced by a woman who has delivered prematurely.

Essence: Breast milk categorised in different terms is a perfect food for baby's initial six months of life

Dos

You have to feed colostrum to your baby as it contains protective substances.

Don'ts

Take the baby off the breast till it is emptied because at the end of the feed comes the hind milk with extra fat which also is necessary for baby to consume.

··18··

WORKING AND BREASTFEEDING

It is not possible for all working nursing mothers to be at home throughout their lactation period. They can continue breastfeeding the baby even after returning to work. Decline in breastfeeding rates across the world has been due to working outside home. Studies show that many working mothers have successfully breastfed their babies.

Going by the guidelines for successful breastfeeding for working mothers, before returning to your work; see that you enjoy sufficient time with your baby, learn to express breast milk, establish enough milk supply by breastfeeding baby frequently and on demand besides practice to give expressed breast milk-feed to your baby with a cup or spoon.

While on joining your work you should take care to breastfeed your baby early in the morning, breastfeed before leaving for work and then again do so immediately when you are back home. If your place happens to be near your residence then try to come back home during breastfeeding breaks. After you return in the evening, you have to breastfeed your baby frequently. At night before you go for sleep, breastfeed the baby as many times as possible, you can also breastfeed your baby as per the schedule if creche facilities are nearby to your place of work. To ensure adequate production of your milk, you can express your breast milk during work in a sterilized container for storage to be given to baby later or discard so as to relieve heaviness.

Essence: Decline in breastfeeding rate across the world has been due to working women

Dos

Learn to express your breast milk to maintain your milk supply if you are working.

Don'ts

Express your milk in a non-sterilised container as it is likely to develop infection for your baby.

19

SLEEPLESS NIGHTS

Most pregnant women go to the toilet during the night, often more than once. Possibly, your baby gently bounces on your bladder to move around during his wakeful times. Instead of going back to bed you start watching TV or reading a book or having some snacks making your baby learn that this is a normal time to wake up.

Also try to learn some relaxation techniques to help you get back to sleep quickly. These techniques will be helpful after baby is born though by then hormones will be released during each feed to make you sleepy.

At the same time you have to take care to see that your baby too gets proper sleep. While feeding your baby, warm some clothing against your skin.

Put the clothing under him like a bottom sheet. This way your baby will go to sleep more easily with warmth that smells like you. Keep the lights very dim. Until about three months, babies do not recognise day or night. Don't talk to him in a loud voice. You can chat with him during day time. Try not to wait for his late evening feed. Make him used to sleeping early so that your sleep is not disturbed.

Babies have different cycles of sleep than mums and dads. After three months sleep cycles of babies change when your baby will fall asleep alone. Some parents want to have their baby in their bedroom but not sharing their bed. They put a small separate cot for the baby beside their bed with its mattress at the same height as their mattress.

Studies show that the breathing of mother and baby are synchronised. If there is a change in baby's breathing, the mother will wake. This is why in hospitals, mothers and babies share the bed. Otherwise also, it is recommended that the mother and baby should sleep in the same bed thereby justify the aforesaid principle of synchronisation of breathing of mother and baby.

Up to six months babies have no awareness and need somebody to take care of them. Gradually, you make your baby sleep alone and shift him to his bedroom. Accordingly, you have to work through your feelings of detachment when it tends to be best for you and your family.

Essence: During pregnancy your baby gently bounces on your bladder because of which you have to go to the toilet often at night

Dos

1) Try to learn relaxation techniques during pregnancy
2) Chat with your baby during day time only.

Don'ts

1) Talk to your baby in a loud voice
2) Make your baby sleep on a separate cot.

••20••

COMPLEMENTARY FEEDING

After the age of six months breast milk only is not sufficient to meet the needs of a growing child. At this time, nutritious solid and semi-solid foods should be gradually introduced in addition to breastfeeding

During the period from 6 to 11 months, infants just learn to eat when they should be given soft foods. You have to see that these foods complement rather than replace breast milk. For grown up infants and toddlers, breast milk is an important source of energy comprising proteins and vitamins. With the result, breast milk has to be continued till the age of two years coupled with the appropriate complementary feeding after six months.

Please note that the complementary food can lead

to malnutrition and also other problems if given too early or too late In case, given too early the infant may not be able to digest the same properly which would increase the risk of diarrhoea and other infections. Early introduction of complementary food reduces the intake of breast milk which is of more nutritive value for the growth of a baby.

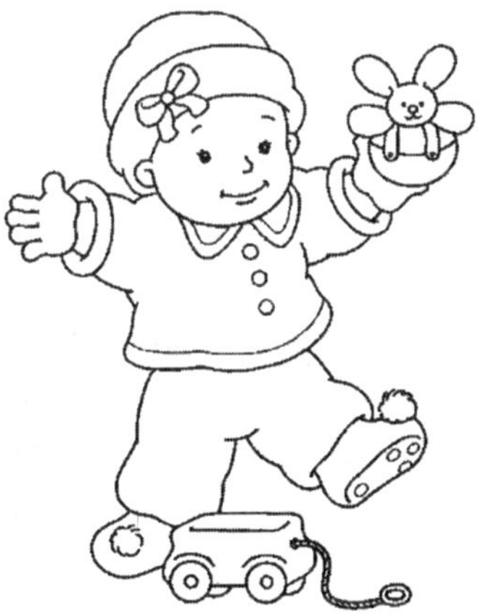

Introduction of the complementary foods too late leads to poor growth with inadequate intake of energy resulting in iron and other deficiencies. The diet should consist of cereals, fruits and vegetables along with continued breastfeeding so as to increase energy intake.

Initially when the complementary feeding is introduced after six months, the baby has a tendency to push solids out of its mouth. So at this time the infants should be given soft and starchy foods based on cereal like suji or fruit like banana mashed. You have to see what the child accepts taste wise.

By nine months of age, the babies should be given chopped foods. With the advancing age of the child the consistency of food has to be switched over to solid food. In the evening the baby may spit out food which should not be considered to be dislike of food.

Coming to guidelines while introducing solid foods, you have to first of all take it easy while feeding your baby and try to introduce only one food at a time. You have to offer homemade family food without spices and chillies. This type of food gives babies a psychological advantage with no need to look separately and its consistency in taste can be modified from time to time.

Continuing with the above tips, commercially processed foods should be avoided as certainly those are not better than homemade food. The child should be served food in a separate plate or bowl that encourages your child to eat by himself besides it will give you an idea of the quantity of food your child has eaten. Never force feed your child. If he doesn't like the dish, give him some other substitute. Don't feed any stale food to your child. Your child needs active feeding which requires your timely attention, interest, love and affection.

Recommended Complementary Foods

The following are common and easily available complementary foods widely accepted for infants.

Cereals: Rice, wheat and jawar are a vital source of

energy providing iron, protein and a certain amount of fat too. Water, milk or milk-water mixture can be added to these cereals to make a thick creamy porridge to be fed to your child. Some oil or sugar can also be put in to help swallowing and making it tasty.

Legumes: These covering lentils, Bengal gram, horse gram, red gram, arhar, rajma, lobia and moong dal are good sources of vitamins, proteins and minerals. With low cost, these are as nutritious as meat, fish and milk when eaten with cereal staples.

Animal Foods: Eggs, meat and fish are rich sources of energy providing easily digestible high quality protein, vitamin B12 and iron. Eggs may be in half boiled, full boiled or mashed form. Meat should be properly cooked and very finely chopped to be given to your child if it falls within your socio-culture beliefs of vegetarianism and budget.

Milk and Milk Products: Milk is the rich source of high quality protein, vitamins and calcium. If your baby is breastfed then he doesn't need extra milk till the age of six months. Sugar or jaggery (gur) can be added to improve the taste providing energy and minerals.

Vegetables and Fruits: These are rich sources of vitamins particularity A, B and C, minerals especially iron and carbohydrates. Vitamin A comes from dark green or yellow vegetables. Potato, sweet potato and colocasia (arbi) are rich in carbohydrates. The same when properly cooked and mashed can be given to your child along with cereals.

Fruits like banana, mango, papaya and peaches provide vitamin A while vitamin C comes from citrus fruits which provide minerals also.

Commercial Complementary Foods

Commercially processed complementary foods are, of course, convenient but are more expensive than family food. These are in no way comparable with home made food. Manufacturers of commercial foods always give misleading information. Moreover, most of these foods are milk based which should not be given to babies up to six months of age. Try to give fresh foods to your baby.

Age related tips for complementary feeding 6-9 months: Breastfeeding is to be continued and semi-solids should be given after breastfeeding. Gradually increase the amount of food. You can also give green leafy vegetables and increase the energy density by adding a little vegetable oil. Feed your baby mashed home made food 2 to 3 times a day for 9 to 12 months: Continue the same including breastfeeding. You can introduce chopped food. In case of baby being a non-vegetarian, fish and minced meat can be added for 12 to 24 months: Continue the breastfeeding. Increase the quantity besides variety. Give sufficient green leafy vegetables. Even if the baby is not well, you have to continue breastfeeding

Essence: Complementary feeding should be introduced after the age of six months because at this time breast milk only is not sufficient to meet the needs of a growing child

Dos

Gradually introduce complementary foods in addition to the breastfeeding after age of six months of your baby

Don'ts

Introduce the complementary feeding too early or too late as both create problems for your baby

21

VARIOUS FEEDING PRACTICES

A baby born has to pass through several levels of feeding such as initial and exclusive breastfeeding followed by complementary feeding.

The first step is to put the baby to breastfeeding within half an hour of birth. This is the time when baby is more alert with strongest suckling reflex. Prompt initiation stimulates breast milk production with better milk flow from mother's breast to the baby. It ensures colostrum providing the infant with anti-bacterial and anti-viral protection besides the crucial nutrition needed at this hour. Timely initiation of breastfeeding has fewer breastfeeding problems with better baby mother relationship. It has been seen that the babies put to breast early have higher core temperatures and less temperature instability.

Coming to exclusive breastfeeding, infants do not need any other food or drink for the initial six months if they are exclusively breastfed. Such babies have less chances of gastrointestinal and respiratory illness including ear infections, asthma and diarrhoea in which case it has a contribution of positive impact on nutrition status of baby while recovering. Additionally, the nursing mother has reduced risk of post-partum bleeding, osteoporosis, breast and ovarian cancer.

Baby's requirements cannot be met with only breast milk after six months. At this time, baby is to be provided complementary foods and fluids along with breast milk. Start of complementary foods earlier than six months replaces breast milk intake which means losing fats, energy and other micronutrients. It is, therefore, recommended to maintain breastfeeding as well as introduction of complementary foods of high nutritive value only after six months.

Essence: Start of complementary foods earlier than six months replaces breast milk intake losing thereby fats, energy and other micronutrients

Dos

Breastfeed your baby within half an hour of his birth so that full advantage of colostrum is availed of.

Don'ts

Give any milk or food in any form to baby before six months of age

••22••

PROSPECTS OF BREASTFEEDING

Breastfeeding is the best way of feeding infants for a number of reasons. It has been seen that even the most careful and streamlined formulae can not replace breast milk which has anti-infective properties. Moreover, breast milk doesn't form a part of any superficial formula. A sufficient supply of breast milk satisfies the entire nutritional needs of infants for at least the initial six months. Easily digestible, it facilitates skin touch therapy that further strengthens the warmth between mother and child.

Breast milk prevents atherosclerosis, hypertension, obesity, allergy to non-specific proteins and develops immunity. Breastfeeding works as an effective contraceptive especially in developing countries where there is not much awareness of latest family planning methods. In India, breastfeeding is the cheap and best way of providing a child a fair chance of survival and good health considering the large majority of poor population.

Studies conducted reveal that the modern woman is less able to lactate with the change of time thereby showing decline in trend of breastfeeding. Education, employment, income and urban residence are the socio-cultural determinants of length of breastfeeding. Most of the mothers say that breast milk is the best food for infants but the actual practice doesn't go by that.

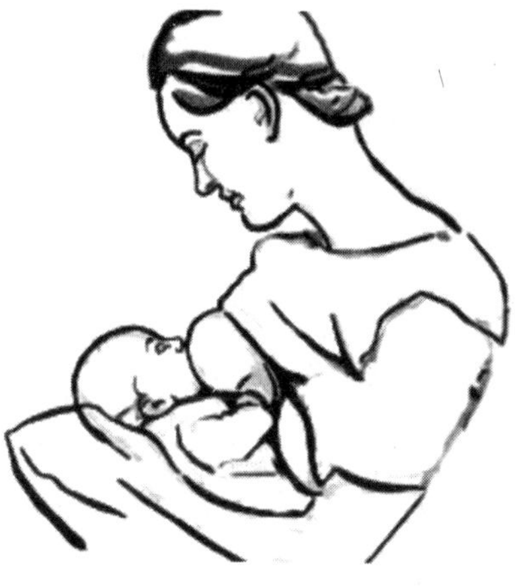

Frequent nursing increases the volume of breast milk whereas less frequent nursing diminishes it. It has been observed that women with normal delivery initiated breastfeeding immediately after delivery. Moreover, mothers who breastfed their babies on demand for longer periods at each sitting could do so successfully.

Even educated women have only partial knowledge

about the composition of breast milk while those who are illiterate are unaware of it. Women working in the organised sector consider breastfeeding as disadvantageous as it affects their figure. A few of them, however, continue to breastfeed for the sake of the child's health and pressure from family elders. It has been neither medically approved nor socially accepted that to stay young and slim avoid breastfeeding.

Breast milk stimulates and strengthens the development of baby's immature immune system resulting in better sound health even for years after breastfeeding has ended. Health care costs are constantly increasing whereas breastfeeding is certainly more economical than any animal or formula milk.

Essence: Women working in organised sectors consider breastfeeding as affecting their figure

Dos

Breastfeed your baby exclusively as it develops baby's immature immune system.

Don'ts

Avoid breastfeeding to stay young and slim as it is not accepted anywhere.

••23••

ATTITUDES TOWARDS BREASTFEEDING

Different people have different opinions about breastfeeding. Rural women of West Bengal say that exclusive breastfeeding is of vital pubic health importance for poor Indian families during initial six months of the life of babies. The advantages of breastfeeding include clean milk supply with excellent nutrients, low cost, enhanced immunity besides protection against viral, bacterial and allergic diseases. It has also psychological and developmental benefits for both mother and child.

There has been undernutrition and recurrent infection with higher infant mortality rates in India due to lack of adequate breastfeeding. Even then many mothers do not opt for exclusive breastfeeding in spite of sincere efforts by several medical and community health organisations. They normally start supplemental feedings too early as mothers feel that the baby is not adequately satisfied with exclusive breastfeeding. It has been observed that the commercial formulas and packed milk products are often associated with communities of higher status.

Moreover, many nursing mothers discard the colostrum part of breast milk saying that it is deleterious to the baby and switch over to animal milk in the initial stage. Some of them consider breastfeeding as too much time consuming. A significant proportion of mothers surveyed are concerned with the adequacy of their breast milk. They were asked to explain as to why their breast milk supply was inadequate. Almost all of them replied that they were prompted to supplement feeding on the advice of some one or because of the baby crying at frequent intervals.

Babies show appropriate weight gain with exclusive breastfeeding when placed under medical supervision. In fact it has been noticed that all episodes of crying of babies indicate hunger responsible mostly due to improper feeding practice. It may be because of inappropriate early supplemental feedings, delayed weaning or excessive breastfeeding especially in the case of some older children.

Taking the extreme case, if there is entire replacement of breastfeeding with cow's milk then it can result in physiological lactation failure with mother's inability to produce adequate quantity of breast milk. The other attitude is of the serious effect of colostrum which is rich in unique immunologic properties important to the newborn. If the colostrum is not given to the baby then it would prove to be harmful because replacing colostrum does not promote normal suckling.

Essence: Breastfeeding has psychological and developmental benefits to both mother and child

Dos

Proclaim the plus points of breastfeeding to all.

Don'ts

Take crying of baby as indication of hunger only; it may be due to improper feeding practice.

••24••

MORE ABOUT BREAST FEEDING

All over medical literature is full of studies regarding breast milk and breastfeeding but in fact very little of the information is actually available to the general public. After the colostrum, the main course of breast milk begins to flow about two to three days after delivery. Breast milk so produced by you contains important vitamins and minerals for your baby including the brain-cell builder taurine. High concentration of taurine in breast milk does seem to indicate a need which can not be met by the child's own body. Cow's milk does not contain any taurine but still high levels of it are found in brains of children indicating it as an important aid to brain growth.

Over ninety five per cent of brain growth occurs by

the age of five years and the same is the average age at which a child is weaned. Two common facts about breast milk are that it has very little iron and it lacks vitamin D but actually breast milk contains sufficient amounts of both the nutrients provided mother takes a balanced diet and boosts her daily caloric intake to around 3500.

Cow's milk contains more iron but that is poorly absorbed by infants. Babies fed with these substitutes get anaemic around six months of age in case they don't receive supplemental iron, whereas it is not true of breastfed infants.

The first two or three weeks of breastfeeding can be difficult for the new mother but later everything becomes comfortable. There are two common misbeliefs that small-breasted women do not produce sufficient milk and because of that reason you can never satisfy your baby's need for nourishment. It is not true. In all pregnant women a physical change occurs in the milk ducts which enlarge the breasts. Moreover, the more your baby nurses, the more milk will be produced by your breasts.

A new baby nurses initially approximately every 1 to 1½ hours. To prevent nipple soreness, try to feed him about 10 minutes alternatively on each of breasts. Gradually the time can be increased. It may take you almost a week for you and your baby to nurse successfully.

Essence: Breast milk contains various vitamins and minerals for your baby including brain-cell builder taurine

Dos

Take a balanced diet to boost your daily caloric intake to around 3500.

Don'ts

Worry as the first two or three weeks of breastfeeding can be difficult for you.

··25··

EXPRESSING BREAST MILK

Many times hand expression of milk is required. Therefore, all mothers should know how to express their breast milk. They can learn it during pregnancy and practice after the baby is born.

Expressing milk is normally required to feed a low birth weight or sick baby, to relieve engorgement or leaking breasts, to maintain milk supply when mother is not well, to leave the milk

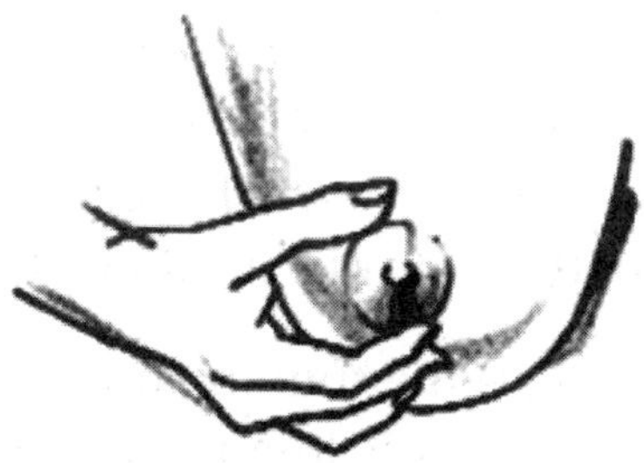

After washing your hands with soap massage your breast for 5-10 minutes with a warm wet towel after which place your thumb and first 2 fingers about 1-2 inches away from the nipple.

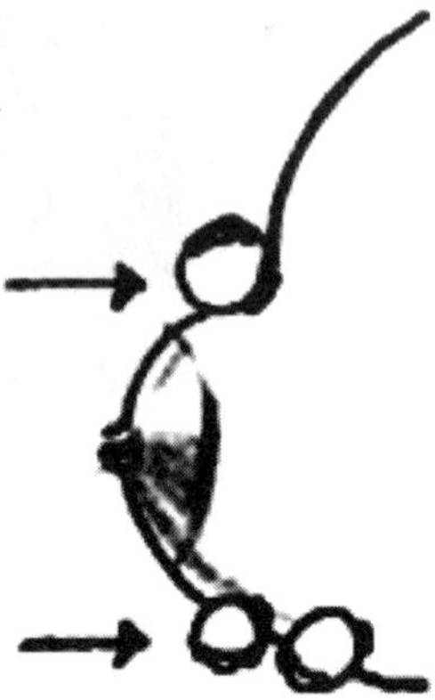

Now push your thumb and fingers back toward your chest.

for baby while going out or to feed a baby as he learns suckling from inverted nipples.

Before expression it is to stimulate the oxytocin reflex to assure better breast milk flow to the baby. Stimulate your nipples by massaging the breasts gently towards the nipple. Stroke the nipple and areola gently with finger tips or gently roll a closed fist over the breast. Do it while sitting in a relaxed mood and manner.

Method of Expression

To express the milk, wash your hands thoroughly. Be in a comfortable position and hold a clean container near the breast. Be confident to take out a warm soothing drink. Stimulate the nipple.

Place the thumb and the index finger on the areola above and below the nipple opposite each other. The thumb and finger should be pressed inwards towards the chest wall. After that the areola behind the nipple should be pressed between the finger and thumb in order that the lactiferous sinuses beneath the areola are compressed.

Pressure should be alternatively applied and released till the flow of milk starts. If it is painful which means that the technique is wrong, then stop sliding the fingers along the skin and the nipple itself should not be squeezed.

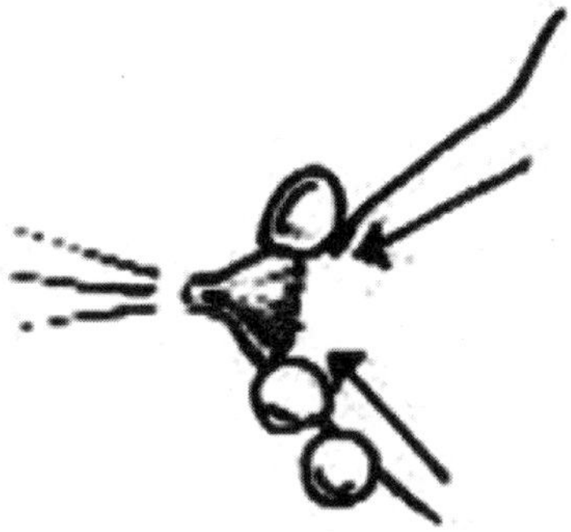

Roll back your thumb and 2 fingers together.

Apply pressure on sides to ensure expression from all segments of breasts. Express the breast for at least three to five minutes when the flow slows and after that express the other breast. So to express the milk sufficiently, it takes 20 to 30 minutes. It is not advisable to attempt expressions in a shorter time.

Breast milk can be stored for 24 hours say in a refrigerator or for eight hours at normal room temperature. Refrigerated breast milk should not be heated because it will destroy protective substances. The same should be brought to room temperature before feeding by a spoon or cup.

Essence: Expressed breast milk can be stored for 24 hours in a refrigerator or for eight hours at normal room temperature. It is not to be heated.

Dos

Learn to express the milk during pregnancy itself.

Don'ts

Boil or heat the expressed milk as it will destroy protective substances.

··26··

YET ANOTHER PREGNANCY AND WEANING

A lot of congrats to you for getting pregnant again which does not mean the end of breastfeeding relationship with your growing child. This is also the time when some babies may be weaned from the breast.

In the early days of your pregnancy, your nipples are quite sensitive and the taste of your milk becomes salty due to the level of particular hormones with the result some babies may temporarily refuse to take the feed. During this period, the amount of milk produced by you decreases. For a few days, you give other fluids to your child till your breast milk supply returns to normalcy. Your baby needs to be breastfed frequently so that your breast milk supply is increased.

Possibly your friends, relatives and professionals in the related field would always advise you to wean your child for fear of miscarriage if you continue to breastfeed. They would also tell you that the quality of your breast milk would deteriorate which would affect the growth and development of the new baby growing in your womb. But all that is wrong. Even during pregnancy, you can continue breastfeeding your baby. There is certainly no harm at all in doing so.

You continue to feed throughout the pregnancy after which you feed your toddler and the new baby together. Such a feeding is termed as tandem feeding. Depending upon the strategy of mothers, they earmark one breast for the toddler or interchange the breasts. This process of breastfeeding creates tenderness between the two babies.

You can always opt to decide to wean any time. you would be advised not to do so until baby turns three months old to enable him to enjoy all important health advantages of human milk. Your milk would always keep on protecting him from illnesses.

In a leisurely way you can start weaning by giving baby other drinks or solid foods. This kind of weaning would be gradually accepted by your baby. He can have one or two feeds a day as long as you are happy in offering them. Your breasts would continue to produce more milk. This slow weaning proves to be best for your breasts and baby's health. If you are to wean quickly and no milk is drained out of your breasts then your breast milk supply would come to an end. Such rapid weaning is not advisable.

Essence: You can become pregnant even during breastfeeding

Dos

Breastfeed both toddler and new born baby frequently by interchanging your breasts so as to produce enough milk.

Don'ts

Be carried away with the rumours of people who would advise you to wean in such a condition due to some or other reason.

··27··

BREASTFEEDING AND SEX

You must have gone through many books and articles on breastfeeding in numerous magazines of medical learning but hardly has breastfeeding been described anywhere as a sexual experience. But still some nursing mothers have the feeling of a deep rooted sexual nature, with the result they are often uneasy and guilty while breastfeeding. It is one of the common causes of failure of breastfeeding.

A psychiatric survey conducted revealed that a few women attain orgasm while breastfeeding. Feelings of sexuality are acceptable within certain limits. To a man, sex means intercourse. Breastfeeding did and still does, perform a vital role as a contraceptive than all the man-made methods put together. This is how families are spaced.

From the age of twelve until menopause, millions of women across the world are either pregnant or lactating during their entire reproductive lives. Breastfeeding makes a woman realize that she is really a woman and it is all because of her hormones. If you are able to understand how a woman's make up revolves around her hormones then only you will be in a better position to know about the success of breastfeeding and its link with sex.

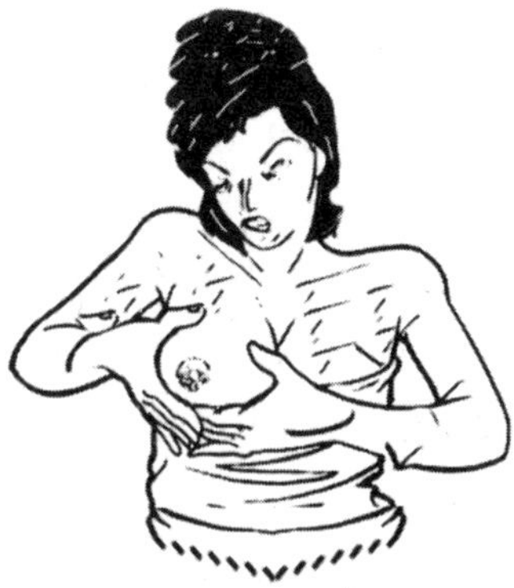

There is tremendous similarity in a woman's periods, pregnancies, orgasms and lactation. In all the cases her breasts become larger because of the behaviour of her hormones on various parts of body in different situations.

Today a woman's breast has a significant role in the eyes of most people and breasts have become the erotic focus for most men as an integral part of the fabric of modern society.

With men emphasizing breasts, it is surprising that sexual vision overtones are often against breastfeeding. It has been seen that many women don't consider breastfeeding with the impression that it will ruin their breasts and so make them look less sexually attractive.

Studies show that many women experience orgasm from breast stimulation alone. Clitoris, uterus and nipples are interconnected by nerves in certain parts of the brain. While breastfeeding, a women gets a sexual feeling at first. Breastfeeding is oftenly a pleasurable experience for women who relate easily to their bodies.

Breastfeeding engenders more positive enjoyable feelings in women and are very much pleasing to their husbands sexually. Actually nursing women return to sexual intercourse soon after the birth of a baby in the case of breastfeeding. Many women are more sexually active while breastfeeding than at any other time.

Take things in a positive way. Show your husband, you still can love. He can even drink your milk if he wants to. This way you can enjoy breastfeeding in the form of sex. Breastfeeding succeeds best in women who like their breasts and enjoy having them touched. Studies have shown that women who failed to breast feed had substantially more sexual hang-ups.

Some women become less sexy while breastfeeding because they feel pain in their breasts and they complain that their nipples don't erect as much as they used to and they lose sexual pleasure. The lactating breast does not swell and thereby the woman feels that she is not responding in the usual way. Another problem is that during sexual intercourse milk from the breasts may leak which some people don't like. So try feeding baby before you make love.

Essence: Many women are more sexually active while breastfeeding than at any other time.

Dos

1) You can enjoy sex during breastfeeding as it works as an active contraceptive
2) You can allow your husband too to drink your breast milk. It would rather help in producing more milk.

Don'ts

1) Think that the breastfeeding will ruin the shape of your breasts
2) Show your husband that you are less sexy because of breastfeeding which in fact can be made more enjoyable.

··28··

MEDICATIONS AND THEIR EFFECT

Most medicines and drugs you consume do transfer into your milk which is often of too low quantity, an order of say one per cent of your dose. It hardly produces any effect on your breastfed baby. A medication reaches your baby after going through various barriers.

It survives the acid in your stomach besides being absorbed into your blood supply, is able to pass from your blood supply into milk, to survive the high acid content of your baby's stomach and be absorbed into your baby's blood supply.

When you are prescribed medicines during breastfeeding, always try to find out information from your doctor or the lactation consultant as regards the medications and mother's milk. Importantly, you have to lessen the amount of a drug entering your milk to reduce the infant's exposure to the medication.

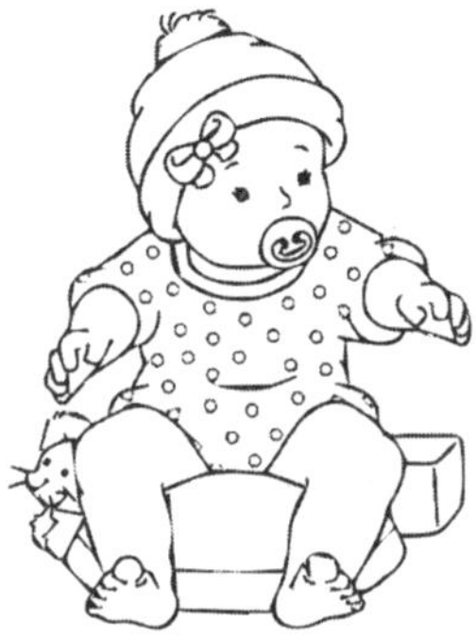

Your baby is not to be unnecessarily exposed to medications and accordingly you have to use menthol steam inhalations in lieu of the anti-histamines or strong decongestants, When you have a head cold, use creams in lieu of tablets for skin irritations and use nasal drops instead of tablets for sinus problems.

Other frequently used drugs are caffeine, nicotine, alcohol and marijuana. Caffeine comes to you through tea, coffee, colas or eating chocolate which may pass to your baby if you consume the excessive amount of some of these.

If you are a habitual smoker, it is better if you smoke after a feed and not in the same room of your baby. It reduces the amount of nicotine your baby consumes through your milk and the air he breathes.

Alcohol has the tendency to enter your milk very easily. While you consume alcohol, your blood alcohol level rises and the level of alcohol in your milk also rises. It normally takes your body one day to break down one standard drink bringing your blood alcohol level to drop to zero. As your blood level drops, your milk alcohol level reduces. Research conducted shows that the babies do not like the taste of alcohol in breast milk and are reluctant to drain the breast.

Cannabis (marijuana) usually is absorbed into fat and stays in your body for a minimum period of one month. It would be important to continue to do this breastfeeding if you have abstained during pregnancy.

All the addictive drugs do penetrate your milk and some remain in your baby's body much more than they do in yours. Possibly it may have legal consequence if the baby is screened for drugs and he may be found to be positive.

Essence: Alcohol has the tendency to enter your milk very easily which passes to your baby. Take care

Dos

Always try to know side effect of any drug you consume because ultimately that passes to your baby through your breast milk.

Don'ts

Consume too much of tea, coffee, colas or chocolates.

29

LACTOSE INTOLERANCE

Lactose is the sugar in milk and is broken down by a chemical called lactose in the baby's digestive system. Babies are usually born with a low level of lactose so that the high level of lactose in human milk can combine with the factor known as bifidus that prevents the growth of damaging bacteria. This extra lactose produces a lot of wind in baby's bowels. You will frequently hear your baby passing wind from its bowels. By the age of six weeks, your baby's lactose levels are enough to break down lactose easily and the discomfort of baby lessens.

Lactose is necessary for brain growth and the babies with congenital lactose intolerance have decreased learning ability. Lactose intolerance may be a problem for a baby after being treated with antibiotics or after diarrhoea. Instead of normal poo, a baby with lactose intolerance will have frothy grey-green poo. The baby will not gain weight and will also be needing the feeds frequently. The baby will cry every time as he has a wet pooey nappy with bottom stings.

This kind of temporary lactose intolerance is treated by using a lactose free formula especially before baby's longest sleep or as an alternative feed i.e. breast for one feed and lactose-free formula for the next feed. In a typical case, to rest the bowels of your baby, give the lactose free formula and then gradually reintroduce breastfeeds.

Some parents assume their children to be lactose intolerant since they are lactose intolerant. In humans, lactose declines at weaning or between three five years of age. Lactose intolerance is abnormal at birth or it can happen during infancy if baby had diarrhoea or was given antibiotics.

Additional lactose taken in by babies causes a lot of wind in their bowels. This excessive wind in turn causes overstretching of bowels called colic because of which babies feel discomfort. It has been seen that a baby with colic may cry for three hours in a day for more than three days in a week or alternatively for a few minutes, Suddenly it may stop then suddenly start again.

Research conducted shows that getting some

support from others is more effective against colic than medication. The use of herbal tea as a treatment for colic is now discouraged. When babies are carried in an upright position, there is no colic discomfort to babies. So carrying baby for a period after each feed any time might help. Hence, all the home grown ways of treatment work in such cases of discomfort to babies.

Essence: Lactose is necessary for brain growth and babies with congenital lactose intolerance have decreased learning ability

Dos

You ignore the sound of passing wind from baby's bowels which normally remains up to six weeks of age. Thereafter the discomfort of baby lessens.

Don'ts

Give additional lactose to your baby which would cause overstretching of bowels due to excessive passing of wind.

··30··

FEEDING ARTIFICIAL MILK

Many nursing mothers choose the cow's milk or powdered milk for feeding their babies artificially which has several disadvantages such as

- it exposes infants to infections because of contamination
- causes digestive problems and malnutrition
- creates suckling difficulties
- does not comprise appropriate amounts of proteins, fats, vitamins and minerals
- enhances baby's risk of developing diabetes and allergic conditions
- does not nurture emotional relationship of mother and child

- has lower scores on intelligence
- does not protect the mother from another pregnancy soon after birth
- does not protect women from risk of breast and ovarian cancers
- is expensive and less nutritious
- is inferior to breastfeeding in all respects

Essence: Feeding artificial milk has no advantage over breastfeeding

Dos

Always discourage your baby from feeding cow's milk or any type of artificial milk

Don'ts

Invite trouble to you or your baby by switching over your baby to artificial milk feeding

••31••

ROLE OF FATHERS

To make your breastfeeding successful, cooperation and help is sought from all members of your family especially your husband who has to play an important role as under:

- He has to make you feel good about your exclusive breastfeeding
- He should appreciate you for setting a good example for mothers in the community by exclusively breastfeeding your baby
- He has to learn about the positive aspects of breastfeeding
- He must spend some time with baby so that you can take rest
- He should help you in many ways so that you can

pay attention to your older children

- He should always make you feel as a good partner and praise your job as a mother.
- He should never doubt your ability to provide enough milk for your baby.
- He should on the contrary help you to produce more breast milk
- He should not feel embarrassed if you are feeding baby outside home
- If he wants to smoke, he should not do that in baby's room
- During breastfeeding the size of your breasts sometimes becomes abnormally large and you are also disfigured for which he should not mind
- He is often deprived of sexual pleasure during your exclusive breastfeeding which he has to bear
- He should always create an atmosphere of harmony at home so that you maintain your peace of mind

Essence: Fathers too can help in stimulating to produce more milk for the baby. They can play the double role

Dos

1) He should always create an atmosphere of harmony at home so that you are able to breastfeed

the baby comfortably

2) He should spend some time with baby so that you can take some rest.

Don'ts

1) He should not smoke in baby's room
2) He should not mind the shape and size of the breasts which get disfigured.

··32··

SOME COMMON PROBLEMS

During exclusive breastfeeding, you usually come across some common problems normally of temporary nature which are sorted out with a little guidance and precautions

In the first few days, when your milk starts coming then it is very important that your breasts are emptied at frequent intervals by the baby so that the same are not overfilled. If your breasts are not emptied properly in time then the milk builds up in the ducts making breasts swollen, lumpy, hard, tense, painful and hot. This is called as engorgement of breasts because of which you feel shivery, thirsty and weepy due to the discomfort. The pain of engorged breasts can be relieved with ice-packs.

Many nursing mothers feel pain in their nipples

particularly in the first week. The peak of nipple soreness occurs on the third day and by the fourth day it is decreasing. The pain is very characteristic and severe as the baby is biting the nipple. When the milk is produced freely towards the end of the first week after birth then there is some fore milk available for the baby. With the result pain in the nipples will reduce because extreme pressure causing damage to the skin by suckling an empty milk reservoir should not occur.

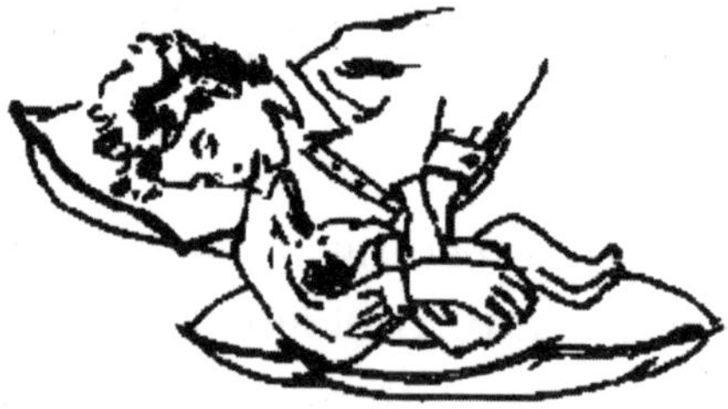

It is very important to make your baby comfortable at the breast so as to avoid this pain.

Some mothers develop a fissure or crack in the nipple normally after the fifth day. It is developed at the base of the nipple and is acutely painful needing careful and prompt treatment. In case the pain is not reducing then the woman may have to put off breastfeeding completely. When the fissure heals then she can gradually resume the breastfeeding.

The problem of a blocked duct too sometimes occurs causing a lump in your breast due to pressure from part of a badly fitting bra or generalised engorgement of the breasts. Milk builds up in the duct behind the blockage and causes a lump. Treatment of a blocked duct should be regarded as urgent as the stagnant milk can easily become infected.

To sort out the blocked duct, make sure the whole breast is emptied completely each time the baby feeds, offer the affected breast first to ensure best possible emptying, gently massage the lump towards the nipple after a feed, check that your bra is not pressing anywhere, vary the position of your baby at each feed, take aspirin to relieve the pain if necessary, make sure you get plenty of rest helping you to feel better.

Poor or delayed treatment of a blocked duct can lead to mastitis which is known as the infection of the breast. Infection develops in the milk that has escaped from the duct into the breast tissue. Its treatment is with the addition of an antibiotic. There is no danger to the baby. You can continue the breastfeeding. Don't be tempted to wean your baby. This sort of mastitis is most often seen after several weeks of breastfeeding.

Epidemic mastitis is another type of infection passed to the breast from the baby causing illness in the first two weeks or so of feeding. The organisms responsible come from the hospital nursery carried in the baby's nose. Many mothers and babies are instantly affected in a hospital. Therefore the same is termed as epidemic mastitis. To take care, a sample of the milk should be examined and accordingly the decision can be taken.

Breast abscess is usually preventable as it follows mastitis that has been poorly treated. Surveys conducted show that such abscesses occurred in women who had stopped feeding when they got mastitis. If the abscess doesn't heal, surgical drainage will be necessary. Don't feed your baby from the affected breast. Simple, carry on with the other breast.

Some babies take the breast comfortably after being born whereas others, however, are completely uninterested and keep on fighting with the breast. This may be because the babies are affected by the mother's pain killers, poor feeding position, inadequate or improper nipples and if the schedule of feeding the baby is disturbed due to the stay in hospital.

A jaundiced baby is often sleepy and finds it difficult to take interest in feeding. Frequent small feeds are best for him. He will develop interest as soon as his jaundice clears. So be patient and retain your milk supply. This may be by expressing after each feed if necessary.

Some babies stick to one breast and refuse the feed from the other breast. So in such cases you express milk from the unused breast to maintain its milk supply. Gradually make him used to taking feeds from both the breasts.

Baby sometimes is overwhelmed by the milk supply that gushes into his mouth. It nearly chokes him. You can, therefore, help him by expressing your milk in a sterilised container and then continue feeding. If necessary, you can also give him the collected milk by spoon afterwards.

Babies who manage to swallow quickly enough to cope with such a fast milk supply may also swallow too much air with the milk thereby developing colic. Some babies in fact bring up almost a whole feed like this. Expressing or just collecting the initial milk should solve this problem. The other way of overcoming the problem of too much is to give one breast per feed. Give the other breast at the next feed.

It is one of the most difficult feeding situations when you have to feed a pre-term baby. Normally, the more immature the baby, the less powerful is the urge to feed. Hence, more of perseverance is required on your part to keep your milk supply till the baby grows large enough to suck strongly.

Some babies are actually born with one or two teeth whereas most of them don't get a tooth for the first six months at least. This would certainly create a problem for you in breastfeeding as baby's gums are not used for feeding. Baby may bite your nipple out of frustration if your breast is too full or if there is not sufficient milk.

Essence: You come across numerous common problems during exclusive breastfeeding which can be sorted out with patience, guidance and care

Dos

Manage to drain out the milk from your breasts either by feeding baby or other means to avoid engorgement.

Don'ts

Wear a bra which is pressing your breasts anywhere causing the blocking of the duct.

33

SOME TYPICAL SITUATIONS

During exclusive breastfeeding you usually come across some special rather specific situations which are to be looked after with the guidance of health care providers and experienced senior members of the family.

Talking about particular situations, baby may be ill or in hospital. Since you have been exclusively breastfeeding your baby, he will not be in a position to recover with cow's milk. If your baby is in hospital, you have to go to him and give him a feed besides skin-to-skin touch therapy. In case direct breastfeeding is not feasible, you can give him your expressed milk with a spoon. You have to be watchful for the baby through out day and night. If the baby keeps on crying then probably he is hungry and needs your feed.

In the first few weeks of life there are many causes for jaundice which baby gets. This makes the baby's skin yellow which may be serious if not treated properly in time. The diagnosis can be confirmed after blood tests. Very rarely a baby develops jaundice from breast milk. It disappears within three to seven days if the baby's breastfeeding is stopped. This type of jaundice is not at all harmful for baby. Breast milk jaundice usually appears at the end of the first week of life. It becomes bad to worst from seventh to tenth day lasting from three weeks to two months.

A jaundiced baby is more drowsy than normal with the result you may have a problem in feeding. Don't allow baby to cry for a long period as it would tire him further. If your milk supply is not enough then give him extra drinks of water to prevent dehydration.

Many nursing mothers with rhesus antibodies in their blood worry if they breast feed fearing that these antibodies may be passed on to the baby through breast milk. In spite of rhesus antibodies in breast milk the same have no effect on the baby as they are not activated in his gut.

If you are unfortunate to discover that your baby has a cleft lip making it difficult to breastfeed, you can, therefore, give him your milk from a specially shaped spoon or bottle.

You have to breastfeed your baby in a normal

way even if he is mentally handicapped. He has to get the same benefits of breastfeeding as other babies do. It would certainly help to bond your emotional relationship with your baby. Gradually, you would be knowing his nature and adjust with him accordingly.

If you yourself are ill at home and you need some one to look after you, baby is to be brought to you for the feed. In case you have to go to the hospital, you have to see whether you can take your baby along. Hospital has to be near your house as someone has to bring the baby to you for the feed or carry your expressed milk to the baby.

Even if you are diabetic, you can breastfeed and feeding makes no difference to your insulin requirements if you eat correspondingly more to make up for the caloric loss in milk. It has been seen that many diabetic mothers feed successfully.

If you had pulmonary tuberculosis and have been free from disease for two years, even then you can feed your baby very safely. If the disease is still active and you are taking anti-tuberculosis drugs, which is food for baby you can continue with breastfeeding

Many babies today are born by caesarian section in which case there is no reason as to why the babies are not to be breastfed successfully. Only due to surgical operation you have a problem in feeding the baby in the normal sitting position with the baby on your lap.

You need to have assistance of a nurse or someone while breastfeeding.

Every drug you take will pass to your breast milk and the same you are feeding to your baby. Many drugs are harmless while others may be harmful even in tiny amounts because of their side effects. If the drug is dangerous for baby then the breastfeeding has to be suspended and it should be resumed as and when you stop taking that drug.

Twin babies demand twice as much milk as one, you will produce enough milk for them. Many mothers have breastfed twins successfully and that too very happily for as long as they wanted to. Don't be carried away by people who say that you have to feed one or both of them any thing other than breast milk. Keep on feeding both the babies frequently and your milk supply would be adequately produced. Irrespective of the size of your breast, you are capable of producing sufficient milk for twins or even more than that if required.

Essence: Irrespective of the size of your breasts, you are capable of producing sufficient milk for twins or even more than that if necessary.

Dos

Give your expressed milk in a spoon to your baby if direct breastfeeding is not possible.

Don'ts

Allow your baby to cry for a long period as it would tire him.

··34··

OUR ANSWERS TO YOUR QUESTIONS

Q. Do I have to drink a lot of milk so as to produce more milk?

Ans. It is absolutely wrong. Sufficient quantity of milk is produced with the adequate consumption of any type of food and fluid by you. The production of breast milk is not dependent on the milk intake of mother. Your baby's suckling on the breast and his frequency of suckling produces more milk

Q. I have small breasts. I am afraid whether I will be able to produce enough milk for my baby?

Ans. Nothing to worry. Successful breastfeeding does not depend on the size of your breasts. The size of breasts is related to the amount of fatty tissue layer under the skin. The breast milk is produced by special glands in the breasts which are present in all women.

Q. Do I have to stop particular foods while I breastfeed?

Ans. No, it is not like that. Even during breastfeeding you can continue to take foods of your choice. In case you have a doubt for a specific food then you can eat it in small quantities. If it doesn't suit your baby, you can avoid it.

Q. It was unfortunate that I was not able to breastfeed my earlier child. It makes me tense that this time too I won't be able to breastfeed successfully. What do you say?

Ans. Don't lose your confidence. You can be very successful in breastfeeding your baby though you were disappointed in your earlier case.

Q. Do I have to eat more during breastfeeding?

Ans. Yes, of course. You have to consume around 560 calories more daily for the sake of your baby. In case you are fairly slim and did not put on any extra fat during pregnancy, you may have to eat even more than that.

Q. When do I have to start breast feeding?

Ans. Breastfeeding is preferably started immediately after the baby is born. As soon as the baby is handed over to you, hold him close to your breasts for skin-to-skin touch therapy which stimulates smooth flow of milk keeping the baby warm as well as helping emotional bonding. At this point of time, start breastfeeding.

Q. Is there any other reason for starting the breastfeeding so early?

Ans. Yes, because during the first hour, baby is most alert and the suckling reflex is most active at that time. Moreover, colostrum is the first yellow secretion from the breasts. It contains substances which protect your baby from getting any infection. Early exclusive breastfeeding prevents breast swelling and pain. It also reduces post delivery bleeding.

Q. What are other advantages of colostrum?

Ans. It has immune properties being actually higher than in milk. Colostrum in baby's stomach and intestines wards off diseases like polio and pneumonia. It helps the baby pass meconium, a tarry substance that accumulates in the intestines. Cells in colostrum called macrophages destroy potentially dangerous bacteria.

Q. Can I breastfeed my baby comfortably if it

happens to be a caesarian-section delivery?

Ans. Yes, you can feed your baby after you are out of the effects of anaesthesia. You can try lying down or in sitting positions in which you are comfortable. Take care that your abdominal muscles are not strained. All mothers of caesarian section deliveries have been very successful in breastfeeding their babies with little support and assistance for the first few days.

Q. I have observed that my baby keeps on crying when I give him feed in the early evening time. Why is it so?

Ans. It has been seen that milk supply is reduced between late afternoons and early evenings. With the result baby doesn't get the satisfaction while taking the feed. To overcome this problem, you have to eat something between your lunch and dinner to produce enough milk for your baby.

Q. Is it harmful to give gripe water to baby?

Ans. Yes, it sometimes contains medications inducing sleep which is not natural.

Q. Which vitamins should I give to my baby?

Ans. Forget about any vitamins or tonics for first six months if your baby is exclusively breastfed.

Q. Please clarify the colour of breast milk. Mine is bluish-white and I am told that it is not rich enough for my baby

Ans. It is normal in your case as colour of breast milk of many mothers is of bluish-white colour. Depending upon its fat content, sometimes you would notice that the colour of your breast milk is different in the beginning and at the end of a feed.

Q. Do babies recognise their mother's milk?

Ans. Babies do recognise their mother's milk on the basis of its taste and smell but they recognise their mother more authentically when they come in contact with the breasts because of skin-to-skin touch therapy.

Q. I find my milk very diluted and thin like water. Is it normal?

Ans. It is very much normal. In the beginning of breastfeed, the fore milk is very thin containing less of fat. While at the end of the feed, it is thicker and so called hind milk is full of fats. Feed the baby in an unrestricted manner so that he gets both. One breast must be emptied out fully after which only the second should be offered. Alternate breasts should be offered at each feed.

Q. Is it possible to breastfeed my preterm baby successfully?

Ans. Yes, you can—no problem at all.

Q. I understand that vegetarian nursing mothers do not produce good quality breast milk. Is it true?

Ans. The breast milk of vegetarians interestingly contains high levels of polyunsaturated fatty acids. Vegetarians do not eat animal foods with the result they are at the risk of being short of vitamin B12 which is essential for normal formation of red blood cells. Hence, the vegetarian mothers must take vitamin B12 both during pregnancy and breastfeeding

Q. How long do I have to continue breastfeeding?

Ans. It has to be continued for a period of six months exclusively and thereafter you can carry on up to two years or beyond if possible.

Q. Often my milk leaks after feeding. How can I stop that?

Ans. It is quite normal and temporary. Just press your elbows firmly against the outer margins of your breasts and your problem is sorted out. Leaking of milk stops immediately.

Q. Is it necessary to take extra vitamin D during breastfeeding?

Ans. Sunshine is the best source of vitamin D than any food. The woman who is pregnant or breastfeeding should get as much sun as she can. Their diet should include vitamin D containing foods like fatty fish, eggs and butter. Vitamin D supplements are available for mothers who have little exposure to sun and are not taking a vitamin D rich diet.

Q. My baby keeps on crying because I don't produce enough milk. What should I do?

Ans. Try to put your baby more often at your breast. Increased frequency of suckling will increase the production of your milk supply.

Q. While breastfeeding I have pain in my nipples. What should I do?

Ans. The treatment for this pain is to feed your baby in correct position. Don't apply any cream or lotion. You can just put a few drops of your own milk over the affected area and allow it to dry.

Q. I am exclusively breastfeeding my baby who is passing frequent loose stools. Is it normal?

Ans. It is very much normal. Nothing to worry.

Q. Sometimes I am sick and taking medicines. Can I continue breastfeeding?

Ans. Yes, even diseases like typhoid, malaria, tuberculosis, jaundice or leprosy don't call for stopping breastfeeding. Most common drugs do not harm babies

Q. Should I wash my breast before and after each feed?

Ans. No, while taking bath avoid applying soap on your nipples. Frequent washing of breast will remove antibacterial lubricating oil produced by special glands of areola.

Q. It is only three months and my baby has started fighting at the breast. Why?

Ans. It seems that your baby is frustrated as you don't have enough milk. Try increasing your milk supply by feeding him as much as you can. Allow him to suck as long as he wants. This way your breasts would be producing more milk making you and your baby happy.

Q. My baby is about four months old. Should I start giving him fruit juices and soups?

Ans. No, not at all. It may prove to be harmful increasing chances of getting diarrhoea and would also deprive your baby of adequate amount of breast milk.

Q. Why is bottle feeding not recommended though I boil the bottles with care?

Ans. Bottle feeding leads to problems such as baby sometimes refuses the breast due to nipple confusion which would reduce your own milk supply. Moreover, in spite of boiling the bottle chances of infection are higher in babies. If necessary bottle should be replaced by cup or spoon.

Q. Can my smoking harm my baby?

Ans. Yes, of course. Smoking reduces your milk supply making your child more prone to respiratory infections and asthma.

Q. How can breastfeeding be started immediately in a hospital?

Ans. Arrange with the staff of the hospital where you are going to deliver. Request them to hand over the baby as soon as he is delivered. Keep the baby with you so long as you stay there.

Q. What should I do if my breasts are full and firm?

Ans. This situation comes when there is delay in

feeding the baby or missing breastfeeds. The same can be relieved by unrestricted feeding to the baby as well as by expressing the milk by hand.

Q. How can one prevent abscess formation?

Ans. In case an abscess develops, it has to be removed surgically. Breastfeeding can be continued from same side even after surgery.

Q. Can I produce enough milk to feed twin babies?

Ans. Yes, no problem. You can easily breastfeed both the babies using one breast for each feed and alternating the breasts for next feeds.

Q. Is there any drug that increases the milk supply?

Ans. There are drugs which have their side effects as well.

Q. What do you mean by exclusive breastfeeding for six months?

Ans. Giving only breast milk to babies during this period without any supplementary fluid, food or milk is termed as exclusive breastfeeding. Research conducted shows that exclusively breastfed babies do not need water even in very hot season. Baby gets enough food and fluids if he passes urine six times in 24 hours

Q. What should I do if my nipples bleed or crack?

Ans. Try to get some expert help as early as possible. Sort out your baby's latching on technique. If it is done, your feeding would be pain free. Your baby's mouth needs to open wide so as to take good mouthful of both the nipple and areola. Go for different feeding positions. You can use a modified lanolin ointment made especially for breastfeeding.

Q. Will my cracked or injured nipples affect my baby? Can I continue breastfeeding?

Ans. Babies usually ignore cracked or injured nipples. They are not affected by the blood in the milk. You can continue with the breastfeeding.

Notes

Notes

Notes

www.goodtimesbooks.com

Have you enjoyed the book?

We hope this book has helped you in

Rediscovering The New World

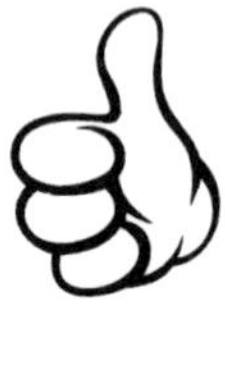